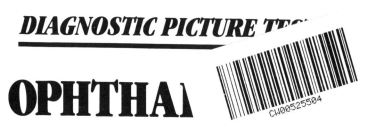

DIAGNOSTIC PICTURE T~

OPHTHA~

Montague Ruben
FRCS (Eng.), DOMS (Eng.)
Honorary Consultant Surgeon,
Moorfields Eye Hospital,
London
Late Professor of Visual Sciences
University of Houston, Texas

Simon Ruben
BSc, MB, BS (London)
Demonstrator in Anatomy
Cambridge University

Wolfe Medical Publications Ltd

Titles in this series, published or being developed, include:

Diagnostic Picture Tests in Paediatrics
Picture Tests in Human Anatomy
Diagnostic Picture Tests in Oral Medicine
Diagnostic Picture Tests in Orthopaedics
Diagnostic Picture Tests in Infectious Diseases
Diagnostic Picture Tests in Dermatology
Diagnostic Picture Tests in Rheumatology
Diagnostic Picture Tests in Obstetrics/Gynaecology
Diagnostic Picture Tests in Clinical Neurology
Diagnostic Picture Tests in Injury in Sport
Diagnostic Picture Tests in Surgery
Diagnostic Picture Tests in General Medicine

Copyright © C. Montague Ruben and Simon Ruben, 1987
Reprinted 1987
Published by Wolfe Medical Publications Ltd, 1987
Printed by W.S. Cowell Ltd, Ipswich, England
ISBN 0-7234-0880-7

For a full list of Wolfe Medical Atlases, plus
forthcoming titles and details of our surgical,
dental and veterinary Atlases, please write to
Wolfe Medical Publications Limited,
Brook House,
2-16 Torrington Place,
London WC1E 7LT

Preface

This is a random selection of illustrations that can be used as a basis for the recognition of eye diseases and does not systematically cover the field of ophthalmology.

In some instances only one answer to the question is possible but in most, the questions can be graded in ascending difficulty. There are a few repetitions of some of the more common conditions where the questions and answers can be placed in a different context. The book is aimed primarily at the postgraduate medical examinee who may not have the opportunity to see, at first hand, many eye disease conditions. We hope that it will also be of help to final year medical students. The trainee optometrist should find it a useful supplement to an ocular pathology course; the trainee ophthalmologist may use it as an introduction to the textbook.

The illustrations are at the clinical level of teaching. The book does not include specialised technical investigations. Most of the transparencies come from the senior author's teaching collection and emanate from the period when he was a consultant at Moorfields Eye Hospital. Some come from the College of Optometry, University of Houston, USA.

Dr Simon Ruben undertook the onerous task of collating the pictures and of doing most of the essential library research.

Acknowledgements

We would like to thank the following contributors:

H. Hamano, Professor of Ophthalmology, University of Osaka, Japan (**107**); G. S. Willetts, Consultant, Ophthalmologist, York General Hospital, England (**96, 97**); David Taylor, Consultant Ophthalmologist, Great Ormand St. Hospital for Children (**27, 79, 94, 149, 167, 213, 221, 225, 226**); A. Bron, Consultant Ophthalmologist & Reader Oxford University, from C. L. Practice, Ruben, Cassell 1975 (**46**); Alec Garner, Professor Inst. of Ophthalmology, London University (**1, 40, 99, 100, 101, 121, 129, 163, 209**); Michael Bedford, Hon. Consultant Ophthalmologist Surgeon, Moorfields Eye Hospital, London (**32, 80, 83, 84, 112, 137, 154, 155, 205**); Emanuel Rosen, Consultant Surgeon, Manchester Eye Hospital, England (**28, 29, 31, 82, 150, 151, 152, 199, 222**); Clive Migdal, Senior Registrar, St. Bartholomew's Hospital, London (**33, 86, 87, 91, 122, 156, 158, 164**); The Audio Visual Department, Institute of Ophthalmology (University of London) especially T. Tarrant for drawing some of the pictures from the Montague Ruben Collection.

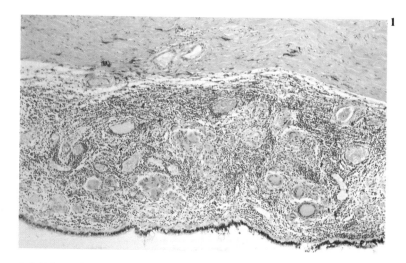

1 (a)Name the tissue involved.
(b)Does this show an inflammatory or tumour response?
(c)What is the condition?

2 (a)Describe the optical system shown.
(b)Is there a practical application?
M=Magnification, Cl=Contact lens, N=normal nodal point.

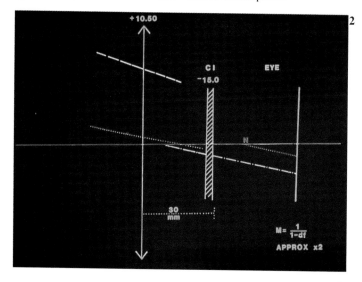

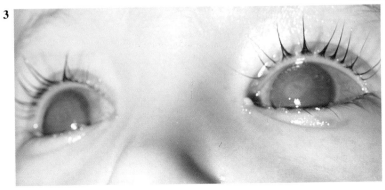

3,4 (a)What abnormality is shown?
(b)What conditions can cause such abnormalities in neonates?

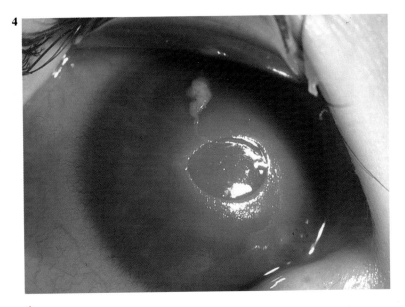

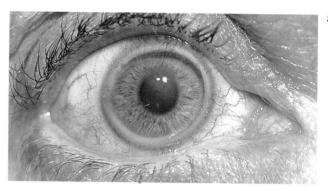

5,6 (a)What is the condition?
(b)How is it treated?
(c)What else can give the appearance of **5**?

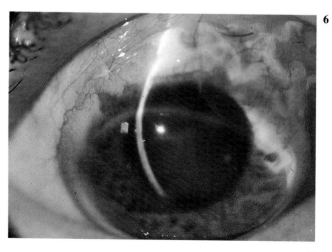

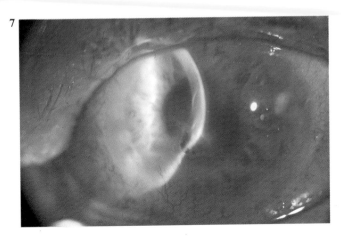

7 (a)Describe this condition.
(b)What is its complication?
(c)What are the underlying causes?

8 (a)What complication has occurred in this keratoconic eye?
(b)What is the cause?
(c)What will be the likely outcome?

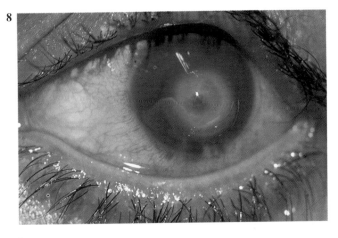

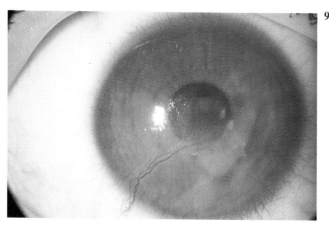

9 A young adult experienced no pain. Schirmer tear test was 3 mm.
(a) What is illustrated?
(b) Which cranial nerves are involved?
(c) How is this treated?

10 (a) Is this Sjögren's syndrome?
(b) What are the ophthalmological manifestations of Sjögren's syndrome?
(c) What are its associations?

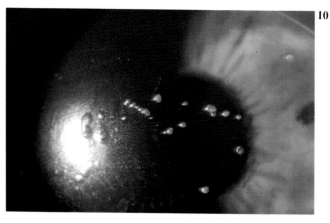

11

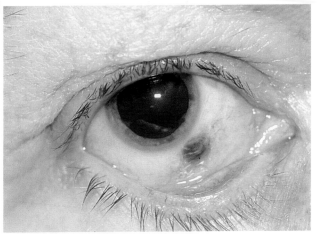

11 (a)What is the most likely diagnosis?
(b)Give a differential diagnosis.
(c)What management is advised for the case shown?

12

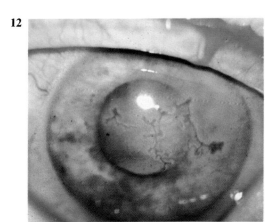

12 (a)Describe what is shown.
(b)Is this a primary or secondary eye mani-festation?
(c)List the pre-keratitis signs and symptoms.

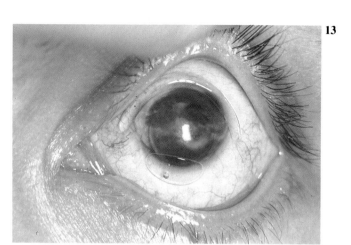

13 A 20-year-old person with a childhood history of eye and systemic problems.
(a)List the ocular signs. Why is the patient wearing a scleral contact lens?
(b)What is the diagnosis?
(c)What else could give these corneal signs?

14 (a)What is shown?
(b)What are likely to be the patient's chief symptoms?

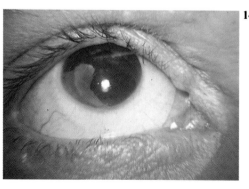

15

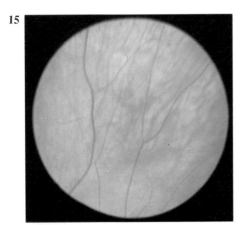

16

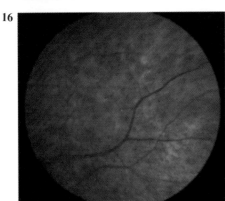

15,16 (a)The fundi shown are genetically linked. What is the diagnosis?
(b)What are the visual abnormalities in each instance?

17

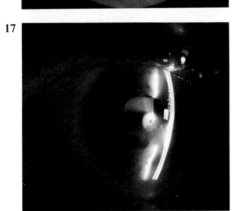

17 The iris has been attached to the cornea from birth.
(a)What is the anomaly? Give a differential diagnosis.
(b)What is the late complication?

12

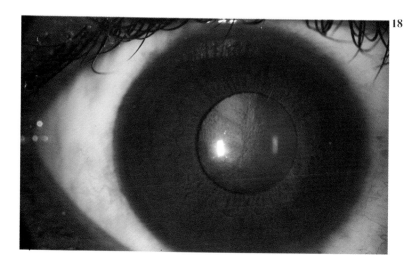

18 (a)What type of cataract is this?
(b)The patient has keratoconus, what is the association?

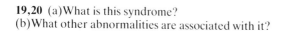

19,20 (a)What is this syndrome?
(b)What other abnormalities are associated with it?

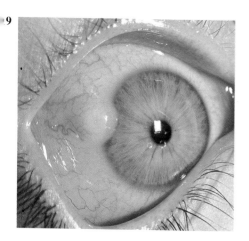 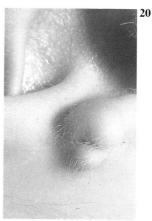

21 This 15-year-old girl has +5.0 (bilateral) hyperopia and sub-normal acuity in this eye.
(a) What is shown?
(b) Is it peripheral or central amblyopia?

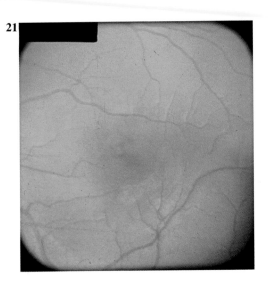

22 The lesion (inferior) is in a keratoconic cornea.
(a) What is it?
(b) With what systemic conditions may keratoconus be associated?
(c) What other eye complications may occur?

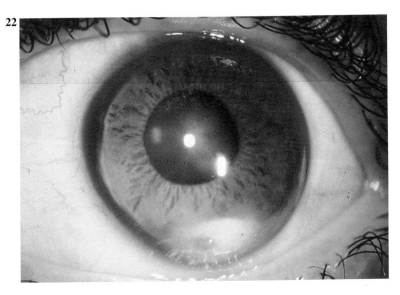

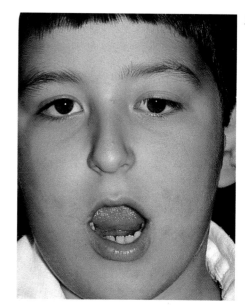

23,24 (a)What is the diagnosis?
(b)Which cranial nerves are involved?
(c)What is the pathogenesis?
(d)What is the prognosis?

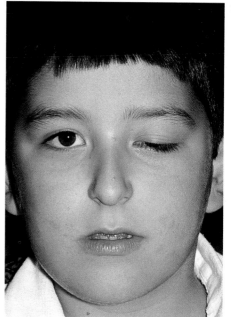

15

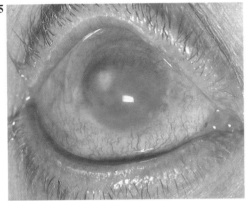

25 A patient from the Middle East. What are the late signs seen and the possible diagnosis?

26 (a)What is shown?
(b)Why is the pathology limited to the palpebral conjunctiva?

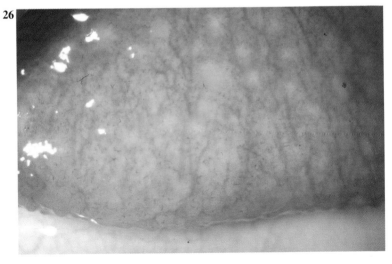

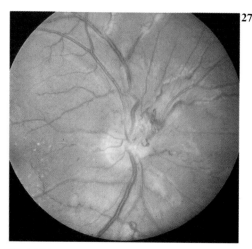

27 (a)List the abnormalities.
(b)Give possible diagnoses.

28 (a)Is this condition congenital or developmental?
(b)Is there likely to be any loss of vision?
(c)Can it change in a lifetime?

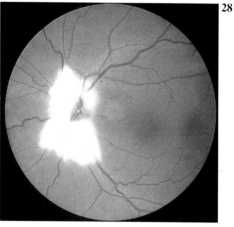

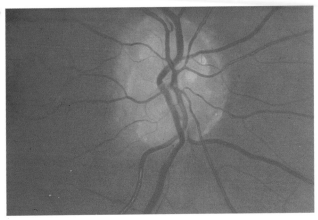

29,30 (a)How are these discs best described?
(b)Give a differential diagnosis and diagnose the pictures shown.
(c)Are there any vision disturbances for **29**?

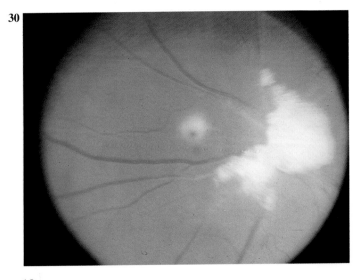

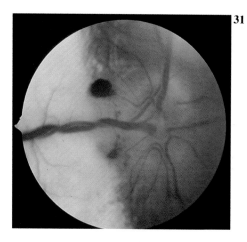

31 (a)List the abnormalities seen.
(b)Why is the chorio-retina blue?

32 This is the fundus of a 58-year-old man.
(a)What is the most likely diagnosis?
(b)Is there any racial variation?
(c)What are the complications?

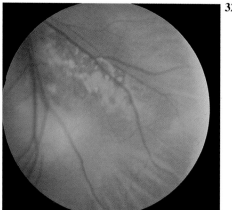

33

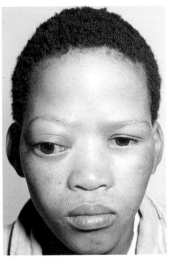

33 (a) A progressive proptosis occurring in the teens. An ultrasound ß scan helped in the diagnosis. What is the diagnosis?
(b) What other causes are there of unilateral proptosis?

34 Sudden onset in a female aged 20 years. It reponded to systemic antibiotics and steroids.
(a) What is the diagnosis?
(b) What is the aetiology?
(c) What are the late complications?

34

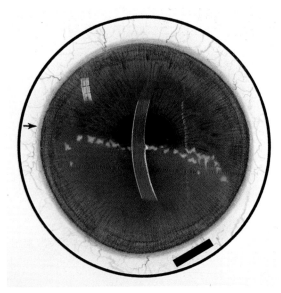

35 (a)What is this tumour?
(b)Does it meta-
stasise?

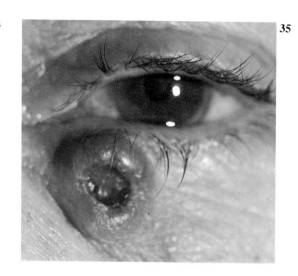

36 (a)What is the metabolic disorder?
(b)List the signs seen in the fundus below, and
(c)others that are associated with this condition.

37 (a)Why does this clear keratoplasty give poor acuity?
(b)What other complications may occur following keratoplasty?

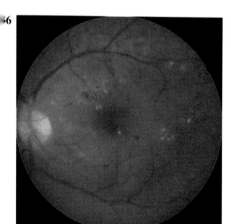

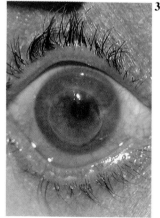

38

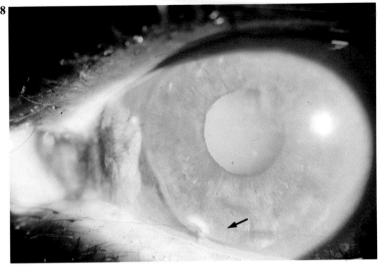

38 (a)What is the abnormality shown by the arrow?
(b)What is the syndrome?

39 A woman aged 41 years, with slow progressive lesion.
(a)What is the diagnosis, and what are the systemic complications?
(b)How is it treated?

39

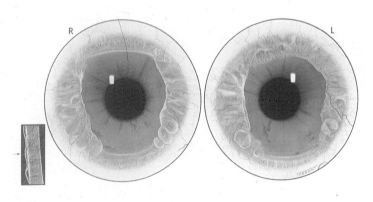

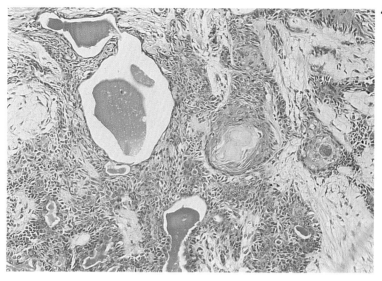

40 Lacrimal gland tissue.
(a) What does it show?
(b) What are the clinical manifestations?

41 (a) Is the pupil natural or artificial?
(b) If artificial, how and why?

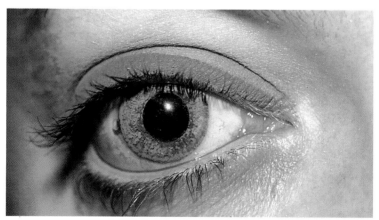

42

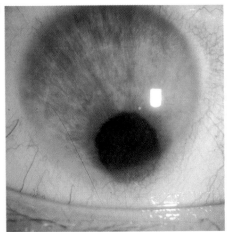

42 (a)Is this bilateral condition congenital or acquired?
(b)If congenital, what may be associated with the eye condition?
(c)What is the treatment in an adult?

43 (a)What type of injury is likely to give this appearance a few hours later?
(b)What is the long-term prognosis?

44 (a)What type of cataract is this?
(b)What is the pathogenesis?
(c)What is the first visual change?

43

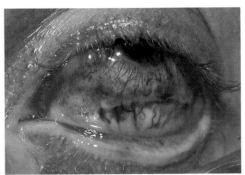

4

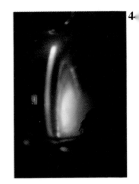

45 This lamellar graft placed in a melting cornea is now itself melting. Why?

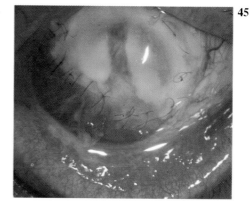

46 (a)What is this abnormality of the corneal epithelium?
(b)What are the symptoms?
(c)What is the visual prognosis?

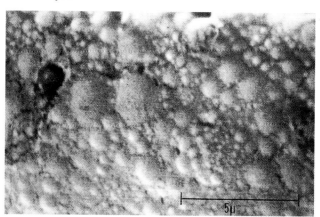

5μ

47 (a)What is the diagnosis?
(b)What other conditions give a pigment deposition?

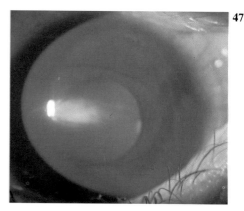

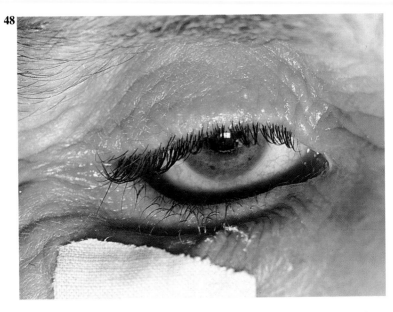

48 (a)What eye complications are associated with facial hemiatrophy?
(b)Name the syndrome associated with this condition.

49 Comment on the disc appearance (patient aged 15 years).

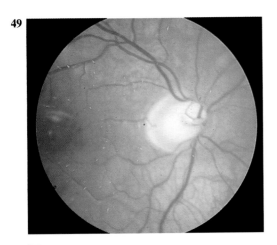

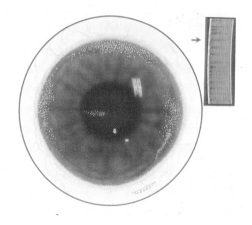

50 What is the significance of localisation in superficial keratitis?

51 What is the keratoplasty complication?

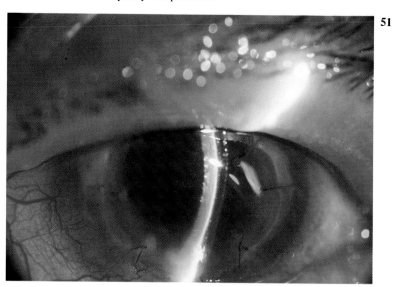

52

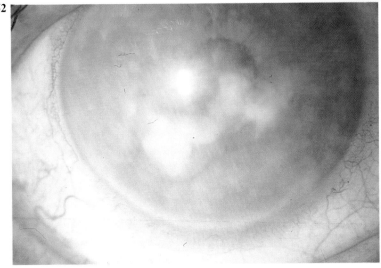

52 (a)Which keratodystrophy is this?
(b)What is its mode of inheritance?

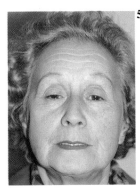

53,54 (a)What is the differential diagnosis?
(b)What tests will aid diagnosis?

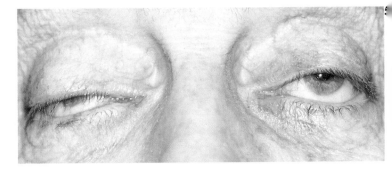

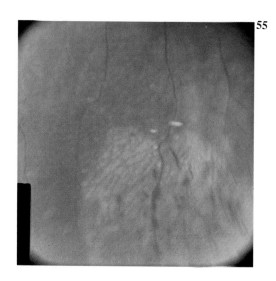

55,56 (a)What is this peripheral retinal lesion noted from infancy (refraction -10.0)?
(b)What are the late complications?
(c)Give a differential diagnosis of the infantile stage.

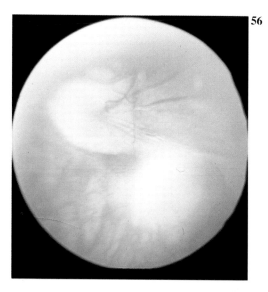

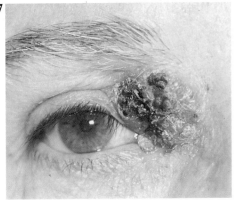

57 (a)What is the diagnosis?
(b)What is the possible aetiology?
(c)What is the treatment?

58 This patient has a history of infection.
(a)What does the picture show?
(b)Give a differential diagnosis.
(c)What laboratory tests would confirm the diagnosis?

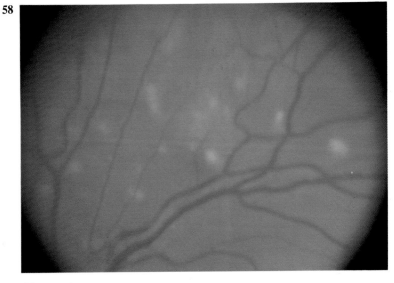

59 A patient with radiation exposure.
(a) What are the early problems?
(b) What are the late eye complications?

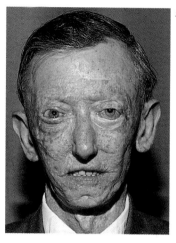

60 (a) Name the conditions shown.
(b) What is the cause?
(c) What are the symptoms?

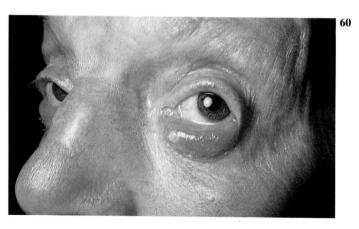

61

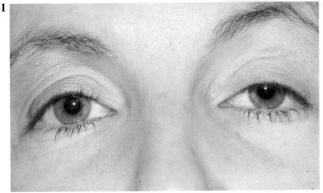

61,62 Why does the left ptosis increase on elevation of the right eye?

62

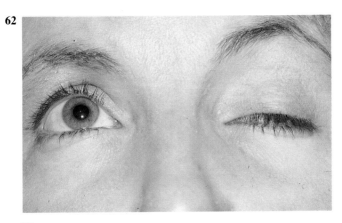

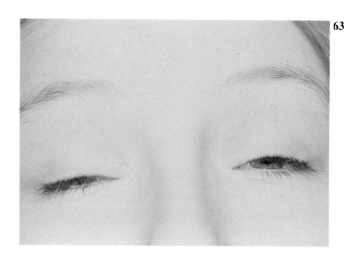

63,64 (a)In this case of hereditary muscular dystrophy (autosomal dominant), how are the lids elevated?
(b)What are the other signs and symptoms associated with myotonic dystrophy?

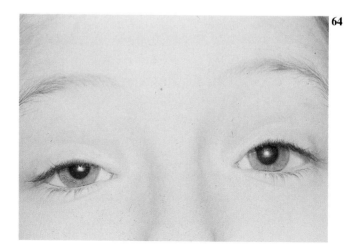

65 (a)What is the name given to this fundus appearance?
(b)Is it a pathological condition?

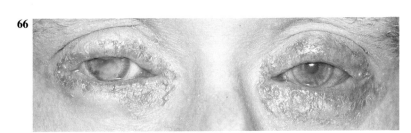

66 (a)What is this condition?
(b)What are the other eye complications of this condition?

67 What anatomical structure is involved in this lesion?

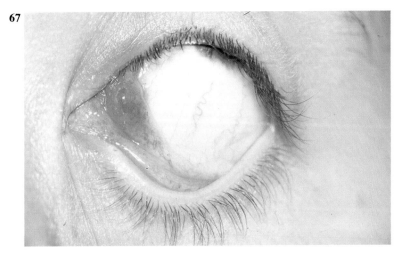

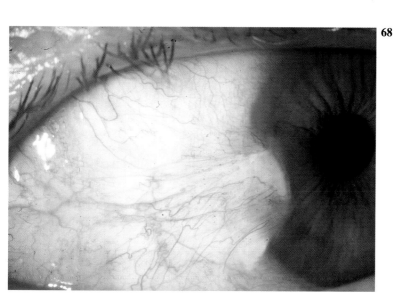

68 (a)Is this true or pseudo-pterygium?
(b)What would the histology show?
(c)How is it best treated?

69 What is the differential diagnosis?

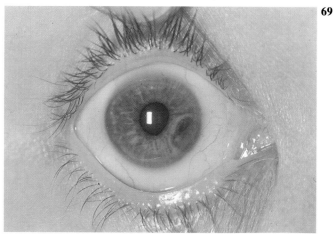

70

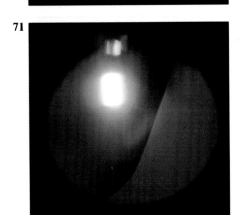

70 The fundus of a man aged 65 years.
(a) Name the condition.
(b) What is the histology?

71

71,72 (a) What is the association between these pictures?
(b) What are the associated symptoms?
(c) What is the mode of inheritance?

72

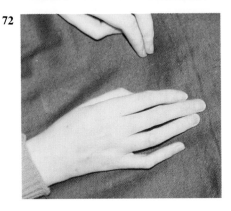

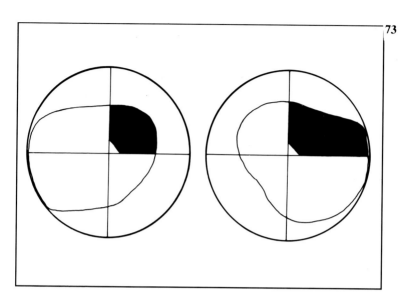

73 (a)What is the site of the intracranial lesion?
(b)What other investigations are advised?

74 The acuity is 6/60 (20/200) when corrected (−4.00 S, −1.00 cyl x180). Why?

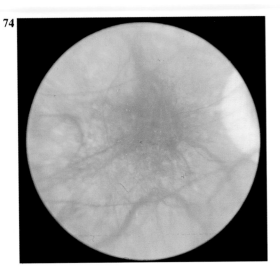

75 (a)What is the diagnosis?
(b)Should local excision or exenteration be performed?

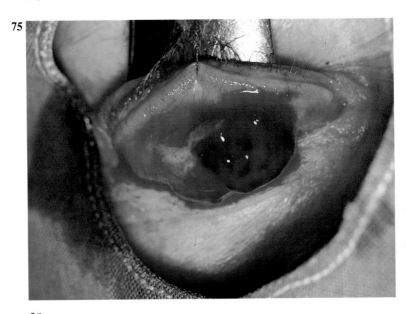

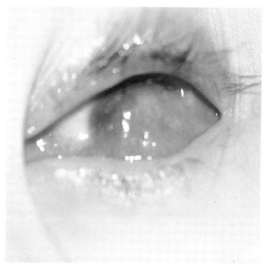

76 What is the most likely cause?

77 (a)What is this infection?
(b)What are the predisposing factors?

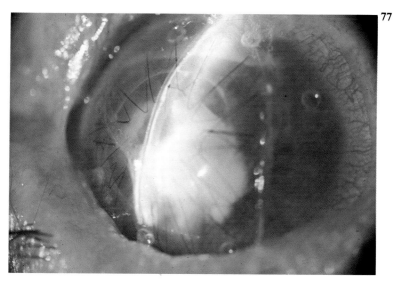

78

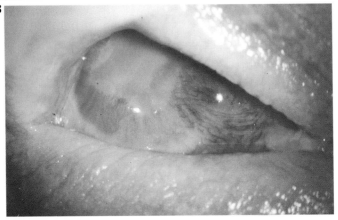

78 (a)Name the hypersensitivity syndrome.
(b)List the most common drugs likely to be a cause of this adverse reaction.

79 (a)Give a differential diagnosis of this type of limbal infiltration.
(b)What confirmatory evidence would help make a diagnosis?

79

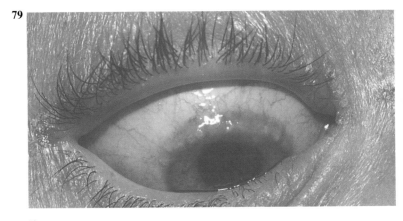

80 (a)Diagnose the disc anomaly.
(b)Is it in the usual position?
(c)What associated pathology can occur?

(Temporal ←)

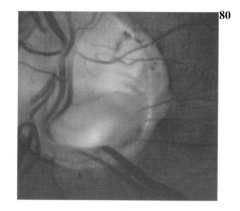

81 A patient with an intracranial tumour. What ocular involvement is shown?

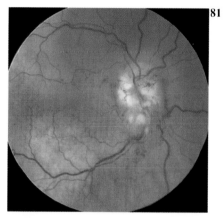

82 (a)What is the C/D ratio?
(b)Is it pathological?
(c)What is the cause, and what other disc abnormalities are found?

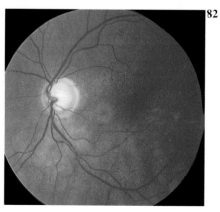

41

83

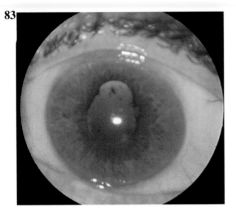

83 (a)What is the cause of the irregular pupil?
(b)List other causes of irregular pupil.

84

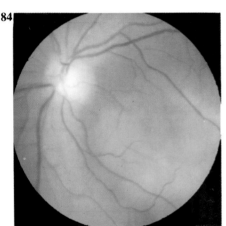

84 What are the most likely primary sites of the choroidal secondaries shown?

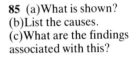

85 (a)What is shown?
(b)List the causes.
(c)What are the findings associated with this?

85

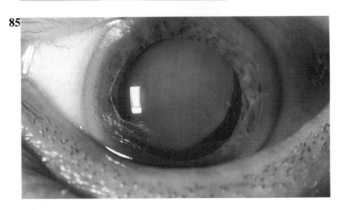

86 A young man. In addition to the eye signs there is a history of arthralgia and urethritis.
(a) What are the eye signs?
(b) What is the differential diagnosis?

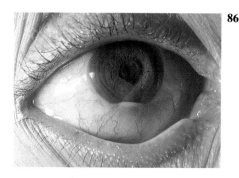

87 (a) What are the white perivascular appearances called?
(b) What is the systemic disease?
(c) What biopsy would prove the diagnosis?
(d) What other ophthalmological findings occur?

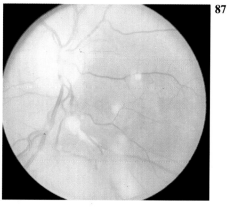

88 (a) What is the name given to this type of keratitis?
(b) What are the possible causes?

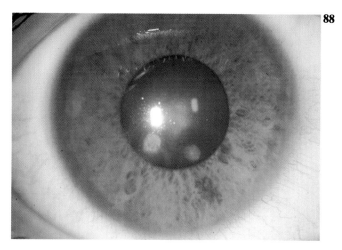

89

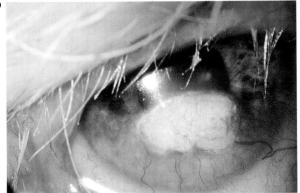

89 What is the lesion seen in this cornea?

90

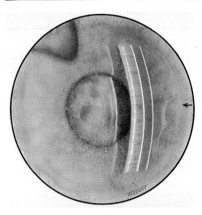

90 (a)What was the operation, and for what condition? (arrow depicts corneal incision).
(b)Is this procedure of any value in any other conditions?

91

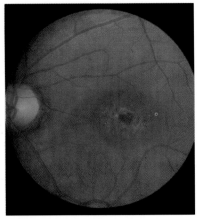

91 (a)What term is used to describe this maculopathy?
(b)Is there an alternative pathology?

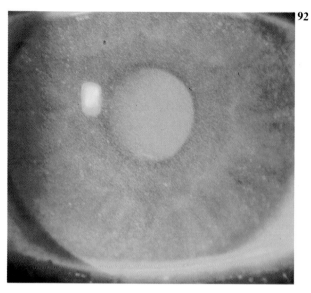

92 What is this superficial keratitis?

93 What operation has been performed?

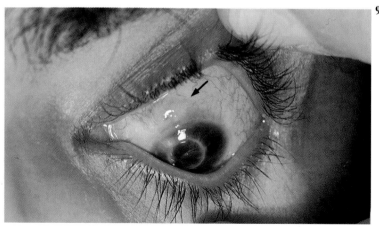

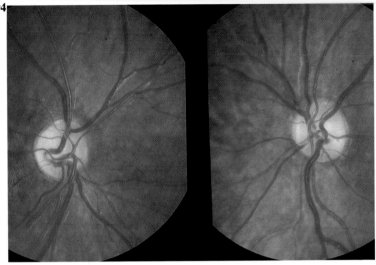

94 A 30-year-old man who has had poor acuity for 10 years. His mother has poor vision and his maternal grandfather was blind from adult age.

(a) What is the diagnosis?

(b) What would the discs look like at the onset of visual loss?

(c) What are the white lines radiating from the disc?

95 (a) Give a differential diagnosis. The endothelial condition is indicated by the arrow.

(b) What is likely to be the epithelial, and stromal state?

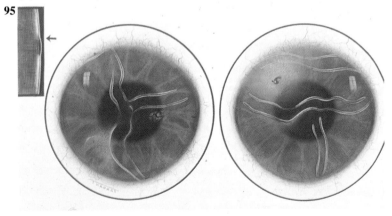

96, 97 (a) Name the worm causing the sub-conjunctival infection.
(b) Name the country and mode of infection.
(c) What may laboratory tests show in the blood?
(d) Is there any chemotherapy?

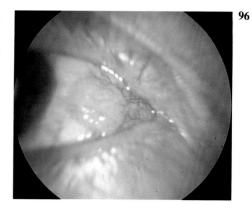

96

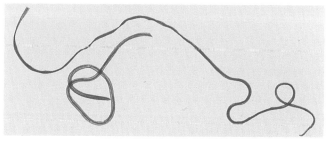

97

98 A patient with a chronic systemic granulomatous infection.
(a) What is the diagnosis?
(b) What are the early and late signs in the cornea and iris? (The picture shows only late signs.)

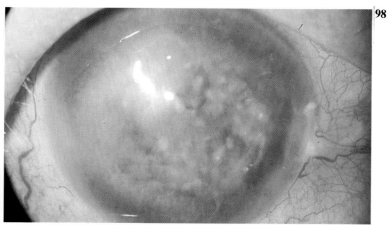

98

99

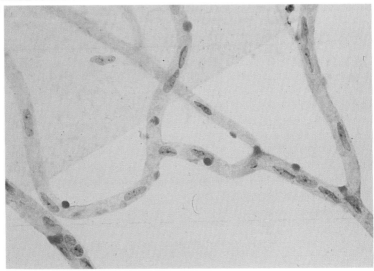

99 A section from a case of diabetic retinopathy.
(a)What does the histology show?
(b)How is the histology represented clinically?

100 (a)What is this tumour?
(b)What feature is shown?
(c)With what chromosomal abnormality may it be associated?

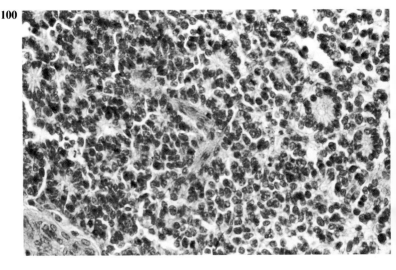

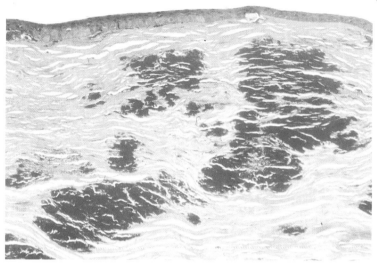

101 (a) What abnormality is shown in this microscopy
section (Masson Trichrome stain)?
(b) Find a clinical picture in this book.

102

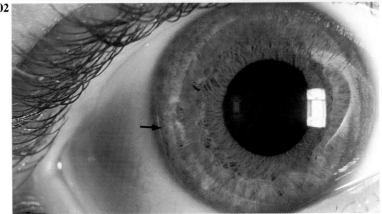

103

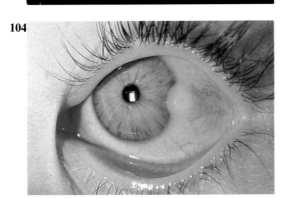

102,103 (a)Is this angle abnormal? (b)Is this related to the white areas seen on the posterior cornea?

104

104 (a)What is this condition? (b)What is the treatment?

(*Left eye*)

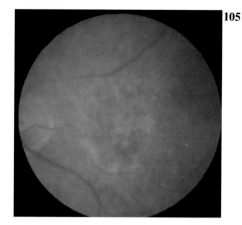

105

105,106 (a)What is the
retinal anomaly?
(b)What are the most likely
symptoms?

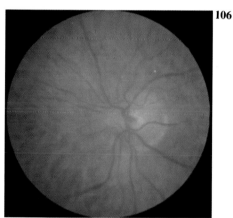

106

(*Right eye*)

107 Could this picture be
seen using routine bio-
microscopy? If so, how?

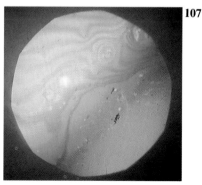

107

108

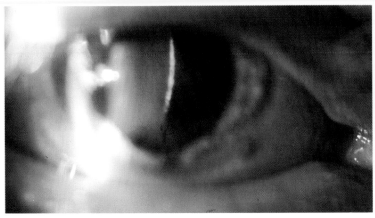

108 In which layer is the abnormality, and what is its significance?

109 (a)What is shown?
(b)Is this condition con-
genital or acquired?
(c)What treatment is
advised?

109

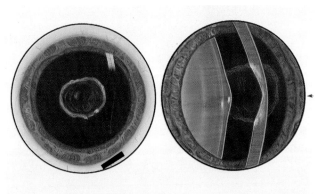

110 Retro-illumination of what?

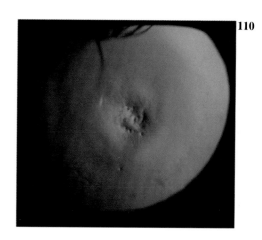

111 (*Clues*: (1) operations during infancy;
(2) patient is a 25-year-old man).
(a) What is the condition?
(b) What is the pathology?

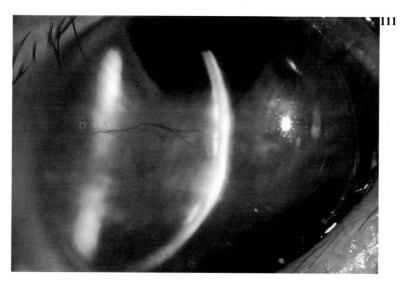

112

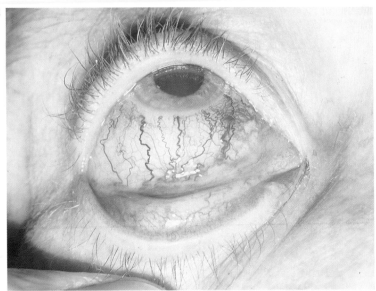

112 Long-standing history of contusion head injury (several months).
(a) What does the illustration show? (only present unilaterally).
(b) Name the syndrome, and the essential signs and symptoms.
(c) What are the anatomical vascular components?
(d) What developmental condition may mimic this disorder?

113

113 (a) What is shown?
(b) What systemic disease could give this fundus appearance in a young person?
(c) Why does this occur?

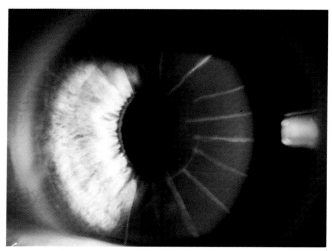

114 (a)What is this operation?
(b)What are the complications?

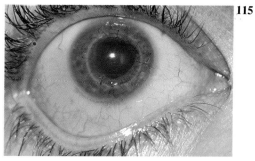

115,116 A patient who has had a keratoplasty and has a fixed pupil.
(a)What else is shown?
(b)Name the syndrome.

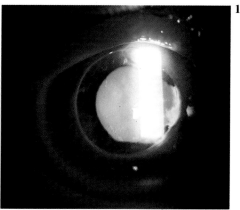

117

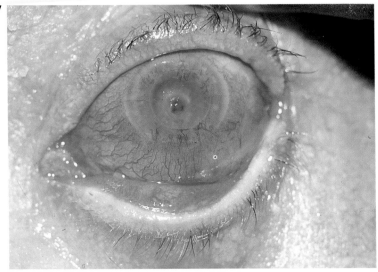

117 (a)What is the pathology of this abnormality?
(b)What is the likely organism?

118 (a)List the eye complications of a severe adverse drug reaction.
(b)Name the syndrome.
(c)Discuss the immunopathology.

118

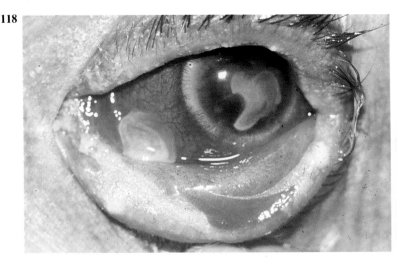

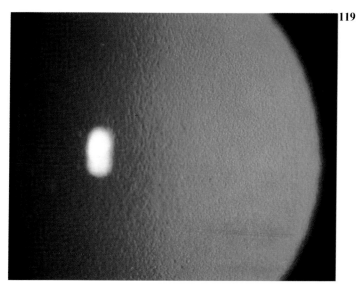

119 (a)What is the significance of the anterior corneal appearance?
(b)List the possible causes.

120 (a) What is shown?
(b) What are the ocular manifestations?
(c) Is there any treatment?
(d) What are the cutaneous consequences?

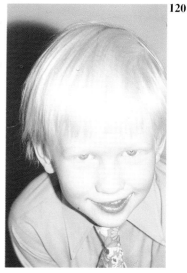

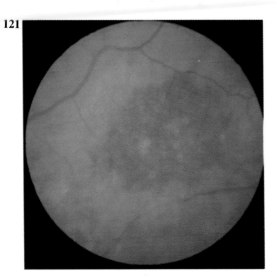

121,122 (a)Give a differential diagnosis of the pigmented area.
(b)Describe the histology.

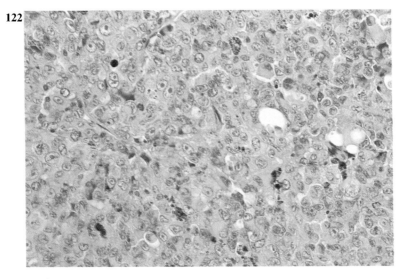

123 (a) What is this condition?
(b) Is it a localised or systemic condition?

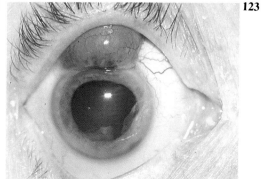

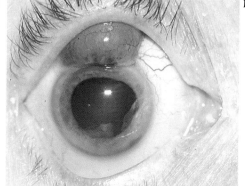

124–126 (a) Name the abnormal signs seen (the illustrations are from one patient).
(b) What is the syndrome?
(c) What is the urinalysis likely to show?
(d) What is the mode of inheritance?

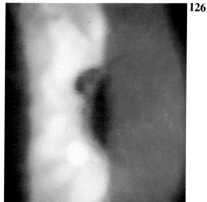

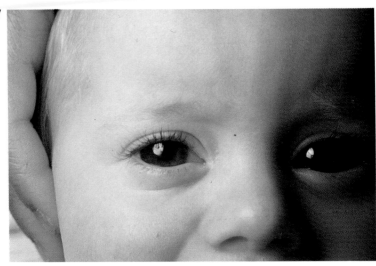

127 What is the differential diagnosis?

128 (a) What is the diagnosis?
(b) Of all eyelid tumours, how common is this?

128

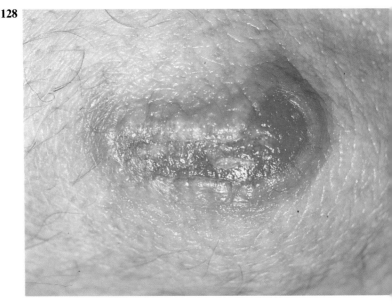

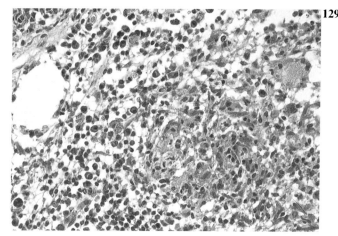

129 What does the histology show?

130 Is this malignant?

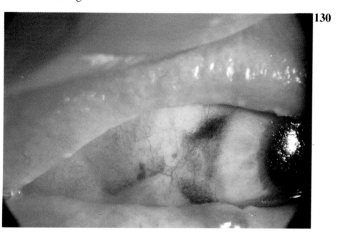

131 (a)Can this congenital condition be bilateral?
(b)What treatment is available?

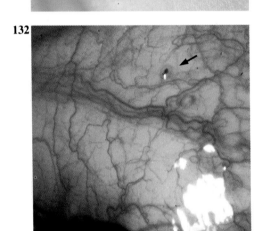

132 Would Sherlock Holmes find this of forensic interest?

133 What was the operation?

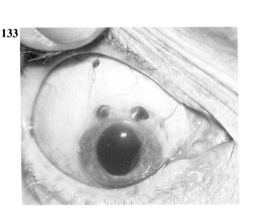

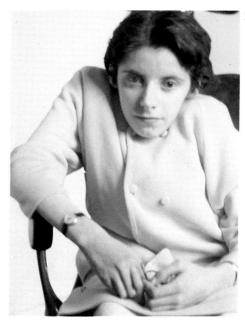

134,135 (a)What is this
bone disease?
(b)What is its mode of
inheritance?
(c)What is its patho-
genesis?
(d)What are its eye
complications?

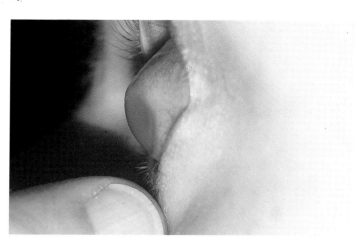

63

136

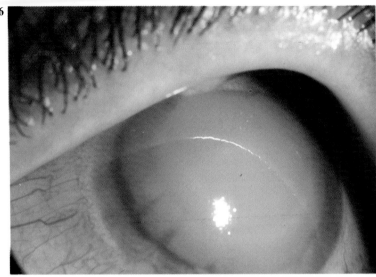

136 (a)What is this?
(b)How did it occur?

137 What is the differential diagnosis?

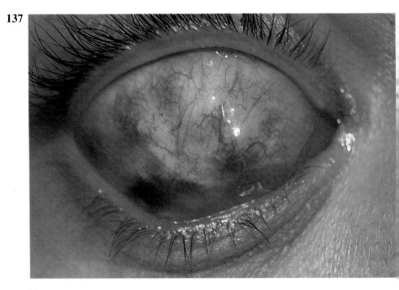

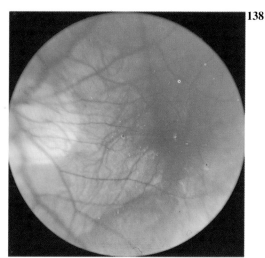

138 (a)What refractive anomaly does this patient have?
(b)What are the posterior segment complications?

139 (a)Where is the lesion?
(b)If the field defect is due to a unilateral space-occupying mass, what could the optic nerve appearances eventually be?

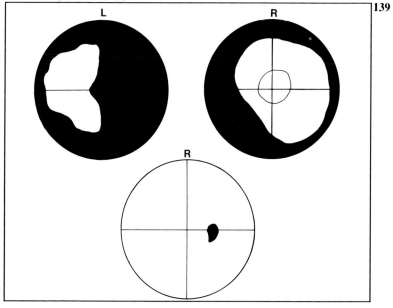

140

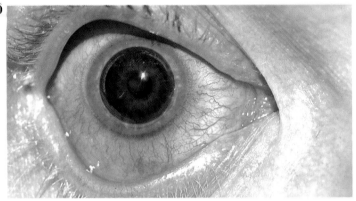

140(a)What is this?
(b)For what is it indicated?
(c)What complications may occur?

141

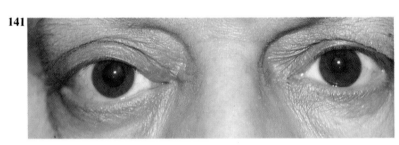

142

141,142 (a)What lid phenomenon is shown, and what is the cause?
(b)Why is there a difference in pupil size?

66

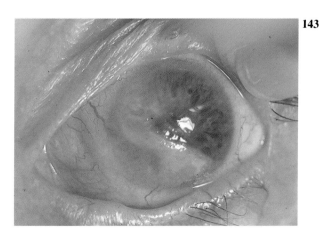

143 A patient with scleroderma.
(a)List the features of the disease.
(b)What are the eye complications?

144 (a)Is this adult young or old?
(b)What would a biopsy of the conjucntiva show?
(c)What is the diagnosis?

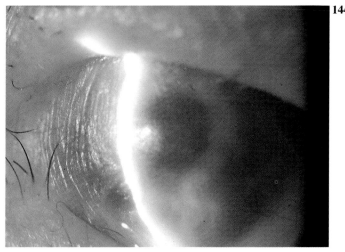

145

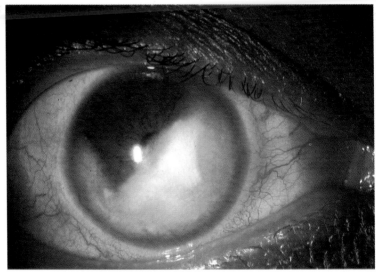

145,146 A patient presented with rapid onset of stromal opacity following episcleritis.
(a)What is the diagnosis?
(b)What is the prognosis?

146

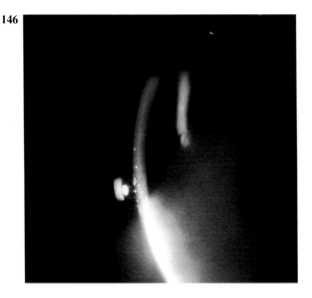

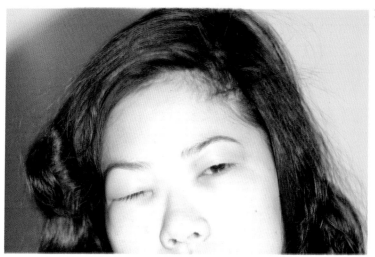

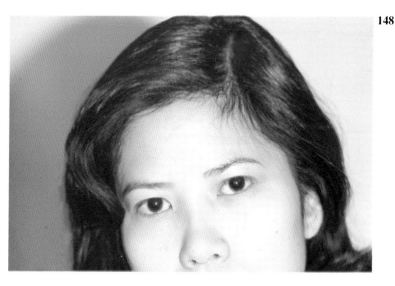

147,148 History was of rapid onset with discomfort, but no eye irritation and normal vision.
(a)What is the diagnosis, and what is the underlying defect?
(b)Name other similar conditions.

149 A patient was born with bilateral Abducens nerve and right facial nerve paresis. What other conditions should be considered?

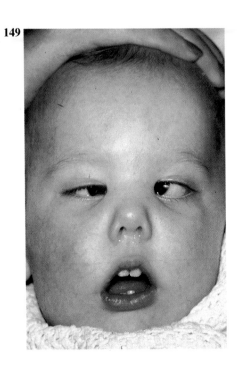

150 What eye tissue is affected by this inflammatory and/or immune response?

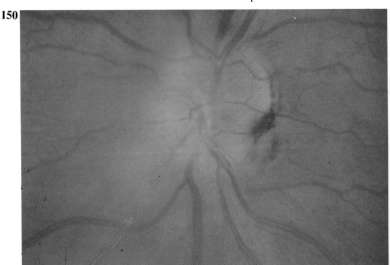

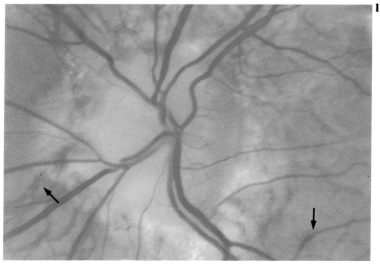

151 (a)What are the bands radiating from the disc?
(b)With what conditions are they associated?

152 A patient who has had a vitrectomy.
(a)What was the complication?
(b)What other complications occur?
(c)What other conditions can give rise to this fundus appearance?

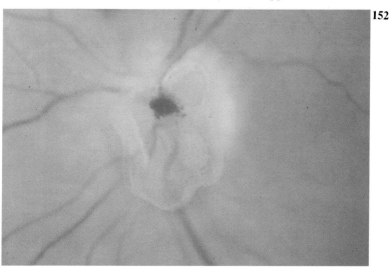

153

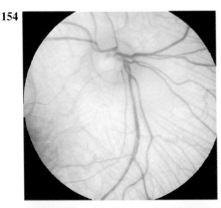

153 Is this congenital or inflammatory?

154–156 (a)Do these pictures show the same pathology, (b)If so, what is the diagnosis? (c)What is the differential diagnosis of the advanced stage?

154

155

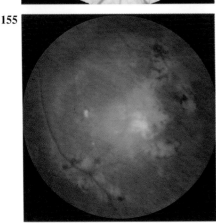

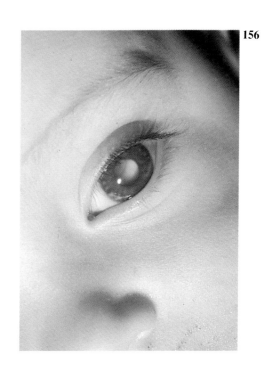

156

157 (a)What is the descriptive term for this disc appearance? (b)What is the underlying cause? (c)What other congenital anomaly may be associated?

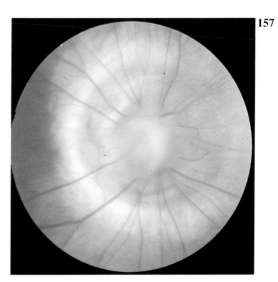

157

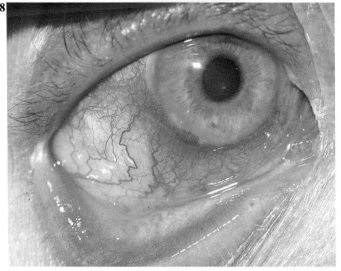

158 What is the association between this, Demodex folliculorum and rhinophyma?

159,160 (a)What have the illustrations in common?
(b)What can be the underlying histopathology of this appearance?

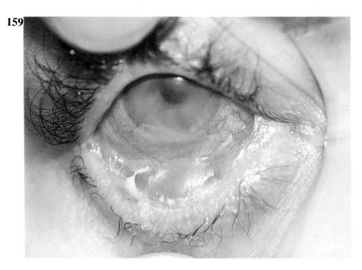

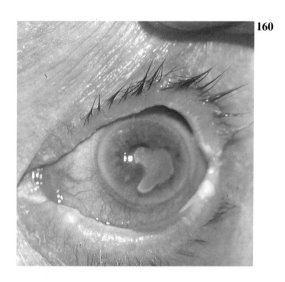

161 (a) What phase of *Herpes simplex* infection is shown here?
(b) What further complications may follow?

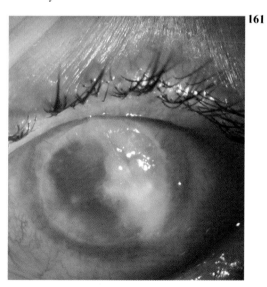

162

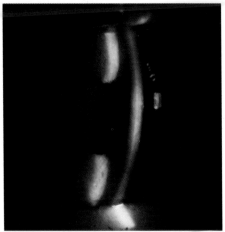

162,163 This patient's elder sister has the same condition and had a penetrating keratoplasty at the age of 55 years.
(a) What is the diagnosis, and what does the histology show?
(b) What measures may be taken to improve symptoms in patients not amenable to surgery?

163

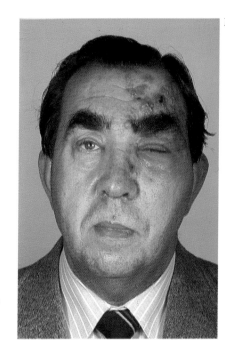

164,165 (a)What is this condition?
(b)List the eye manifestations of this condition.

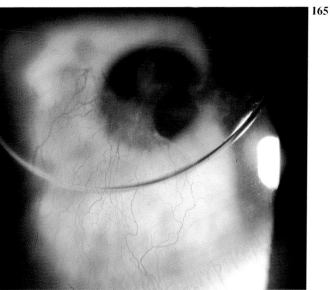

77

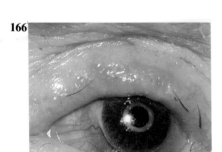

166 What is this operation, and for what condition is it used?

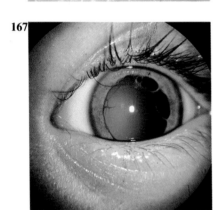

167 (a)Is the pupil pathological?
(b)What are the symptoms?

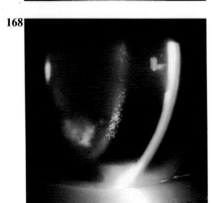

168 (a)What is shown here?
(b)Is this a normal phenomenon?
(c)What is their origin?

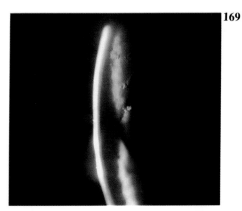

169,170 After thyroidectomy this patient developed cataract and corneal signs. Why?

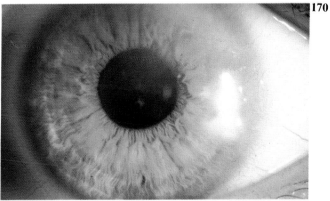

171 (a) What is the diagnosis?
(b) What is the underlying aetiology?

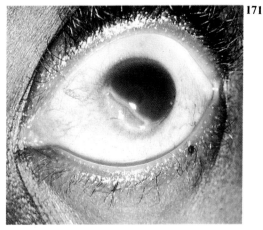

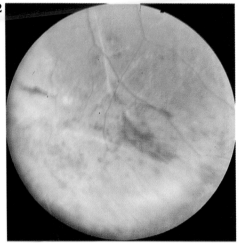

172 (a)What is the inferior area likely to be?
(b)List some common causes.

173 In which corneal layer is the anomaly indicated by the arrow?

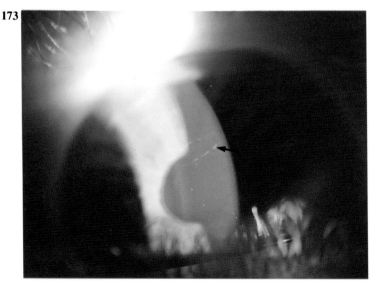

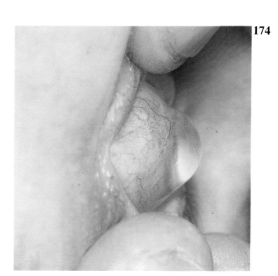

174 (a)What is the diagnosis?
(b)Is any surgical intervention indicated?

175 Is this fundus anomaly inflammatory or congenital in aetiology?

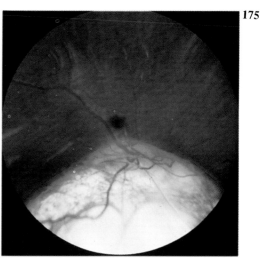

176

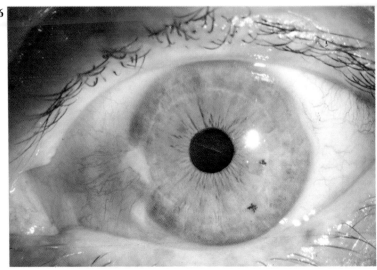

176 (a) What is illustrated?
(b) What is the aetiology of this condition?

177

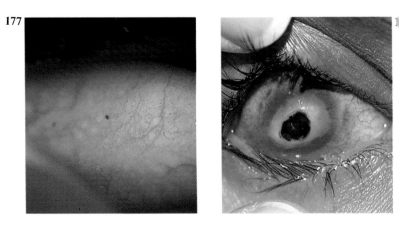

177 (a) What are the black spots on the tarsal conjunctiva?
(b) What other causes of conjunctival pigmentation occur?

178 What is the black area on the cornea?

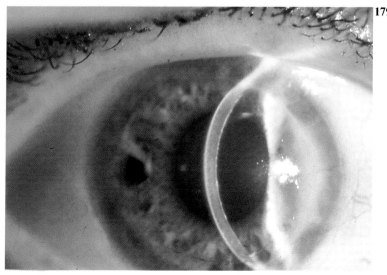

179 What is the abnormality in this penetrating keratoplasty?

180 (a)Which cranial nerve is involved?
(b)What is the eye complication?

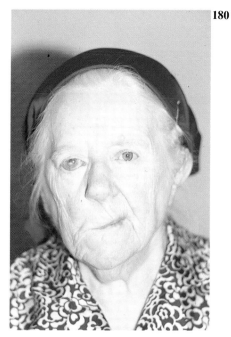

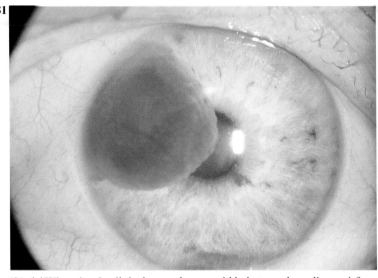

181 (a)What simple clinical procedure would help to make a diagnosis?
(b)What might the diagnosis be?

182 Give a differential diagnosis.

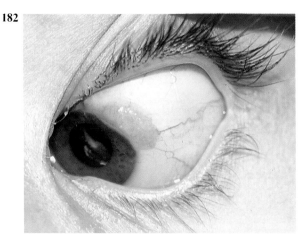

84

183 This condition was first diagnosed at the age of 8 years.
(a)What is the diagnosis?
(b)What are the presenting features?
(c)What diagnostic tests are useful?

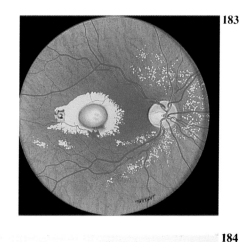

183

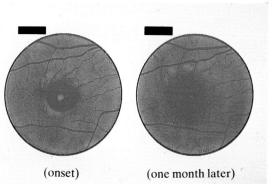

184

(onset)   (one month later)

184 (a)What is this condition?
(b)What is the prognosis?
(c)How is it treated?

185 This retinal condition received no treatment. What was the original diagnosis?

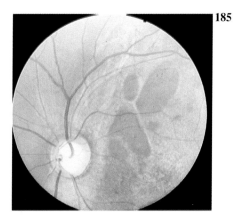

185

85

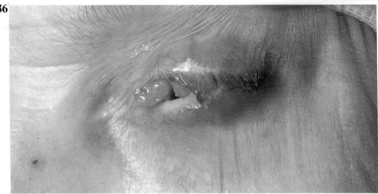

186 What is the neoplasm/tumour?

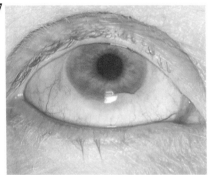

187 (a)What is shown?
(b)Is it a pathological condition?

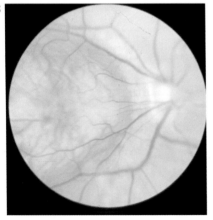

188 (a)What type of injury causes this picture?
(b)What is it called?
(c)Where is the site of the pathology?

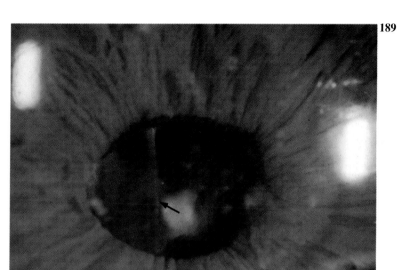

189 (a) What are the opacities seen in the anterior chamber?
(b) What does the arrow indicate?
(c) What visual effects occur?
(d) Of what do these opacities consist?

190 List the possible causes of orbital tumour in the first few months of life.

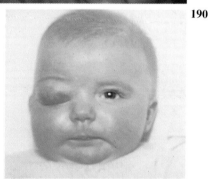

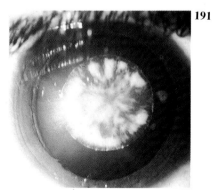

191 (a) What type of cataract is this?
(b) Is it hereditary?

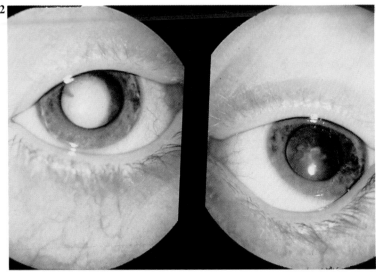

192 A pupil soon after birth.
(a)What is the aetiology?
(b)What are the other features associated with this?

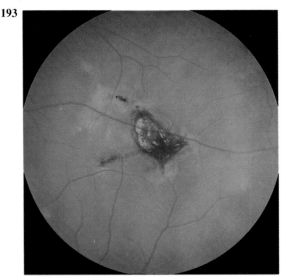

193 (a)What is the infection?
(b)What does the picture show?
(c)What other clinical syndromes occur with this infection?

194 (a)What is this condition?
(b)Name some of the associated disorders.

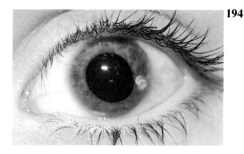

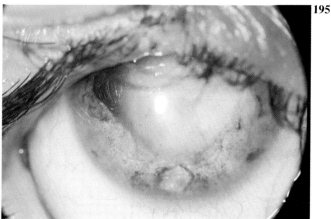

195 What is the cause of the cataract?

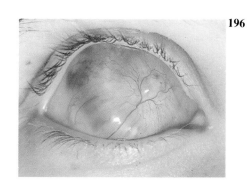

196 (a)What is the condition and probable aetiology?
(b)List possible changes with time.

197

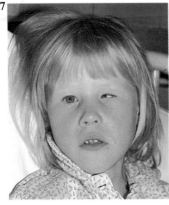

197 (a)Name the anomaly.
(b)What is the aetiology?
(c)Name the treatment.

198

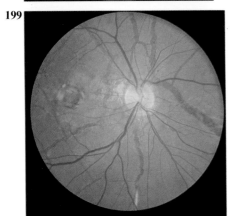

198 (a)List the abnormal signs.
(b)What is the diagnosis?

199

199 (a)List the retinal anomalies.
(b)What are the possible diagnose

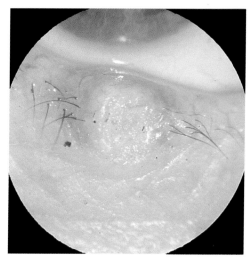

200 What is the histology of this clinical condition?

201 (a)What is the diagnosis?
(b)List the changes shown.

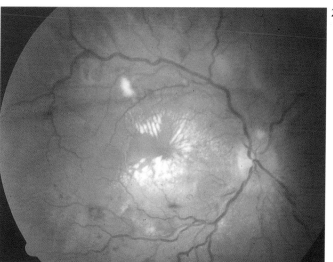

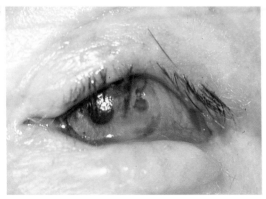

202 What corneal pathology is shown, and why has it occurred?

203 What is the spot diagnosis?

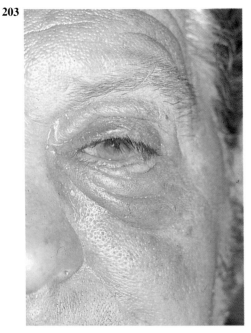

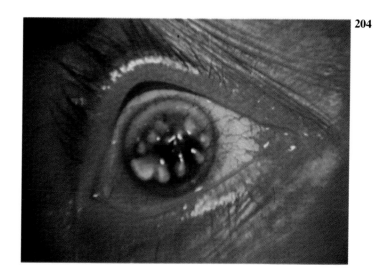

204 (a)Name the condition.
(b)Is it a primary or secondary condition?

205 This is not a squamous cell carcinoma. What is it?

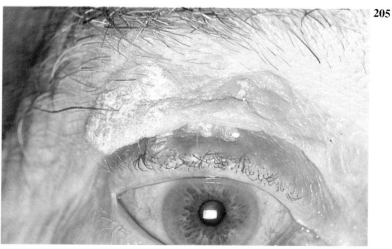

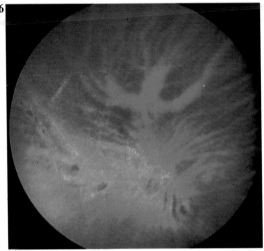

206 (a)What type of retinal degeneration is this?
(b)What type of refractive condition is commonly associated?

207 What is this anterior corneal keratodystrophy and its mode of inheritance?

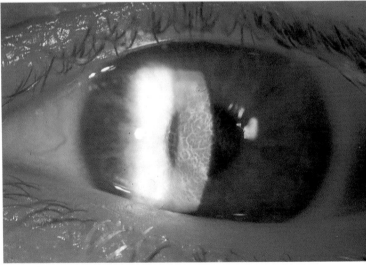

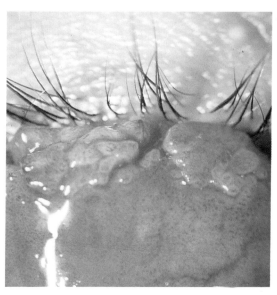

208,209 (a)What does this section from a conjunctival biopsy show?
(b)What other condition simulates the clinical picture illustrated?

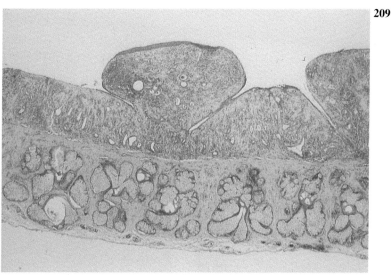

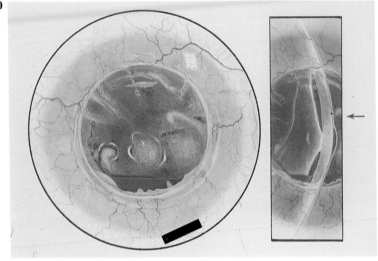

210 List the pathological features.

211 Give a diagnosis of the abnormalities seen.

212 What is this retinal pigment line?

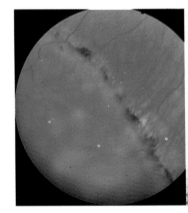

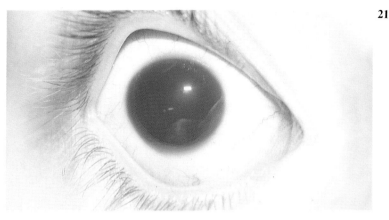

213,214 (a)Is this congenital or traumatic aniridia?
(b)What is the late complication?

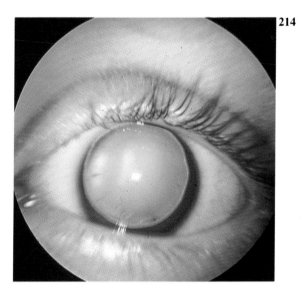

215

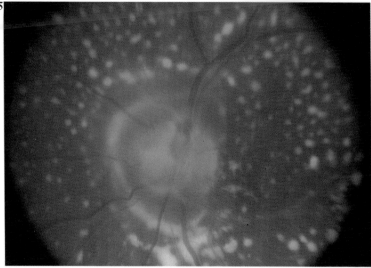

215 (a)Give a possible diagnosis and symptoms.
(b)What well known retinopathy gives the same clinical symptoms?
(c)Suggest diagnostic tests.

216 What effect does an oval graft with the long axis at 90° have upon astigmatism?

216

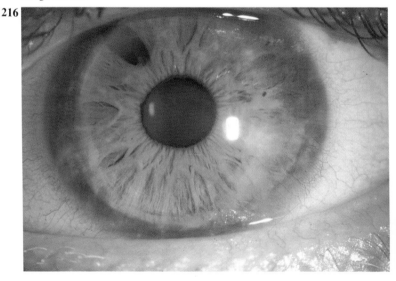

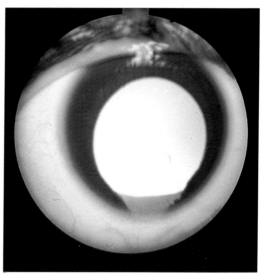

217,218 Are these conditions associated?

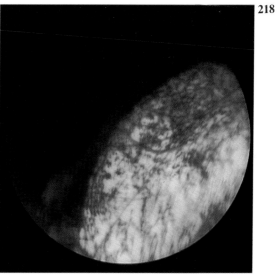

219

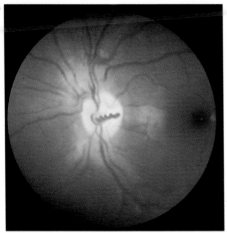

219 This vessel is in the vitreous. What is it?

220 Is there an abnormality of the fundus?

220

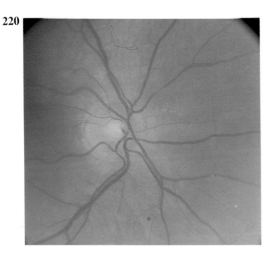

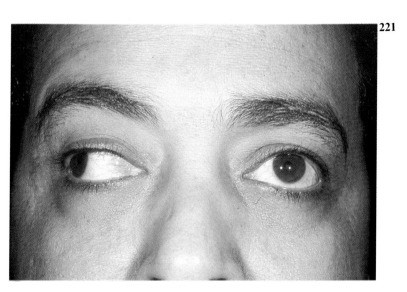

221 An adult presented with rapid onset of paresis of right adduction with a left nystagmus.
(a) What is the site of the lesion?
(b) What is the probable diagnosis?

222 A diabetic patient. What is the retinal complication shown?

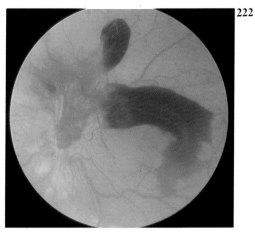

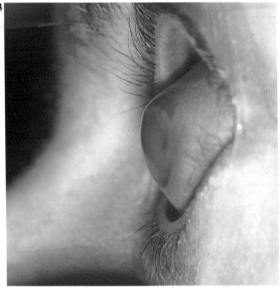

223 (a)What is the diagnosis based upon the scleral appearance?
(b)What is the differential diagnosis?

224 (a)Comment on the pupil size differences: a cryptic answer would be likely to give a false impression in any light.
(b)List the neurological causes of pupil inequality.

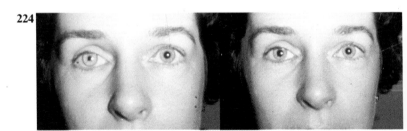

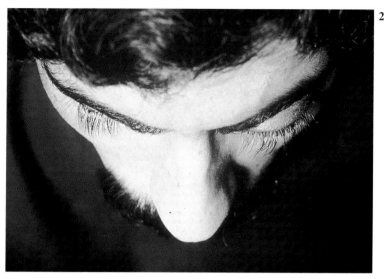

225,226 This 43-year-old has a retro-ocular tumour. List the possible general causes of unilateral proptosis.

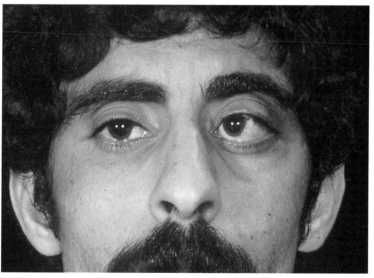

227

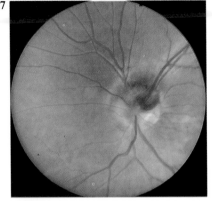

228

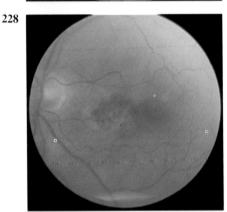

227,228 Are these pigmentary lesions benign or malignant?

229

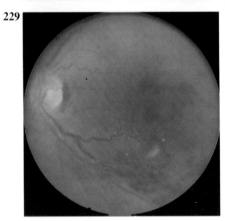

229 (a) What type of retinopathy is shown?
(b) Describe a classification of degrees of severity.
(c) What grade does this picture show?

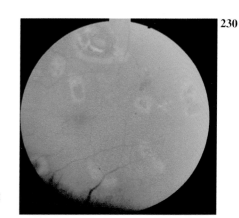

230

230, 231 (a) What treatment has this patient had?
(b) Why has a green filter been used?

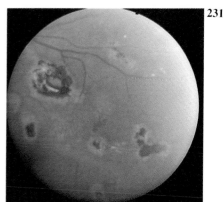

231

232 (a) What is the origin of this condition?
(b) Can it be treated?

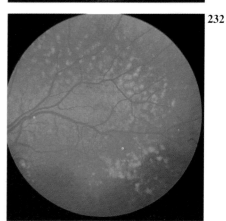

232

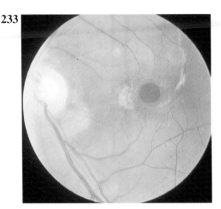

233 This condition has a predilection for males from early infancy to young adulthood. What is it?

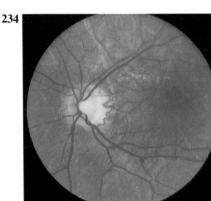

234 This rare condition affects children more frequently than adults.
(a) What is this condition?
(b) Why are children more susceptible?

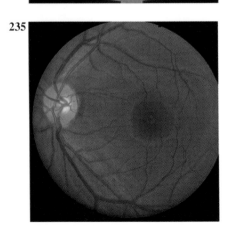

235 What is the cause of this fundus appearance?

236 (a)What is this tumour?
(b)What is the likelihood of systemic involvement?
(c)Give a differential diagnosis if proptosis is *also* present.

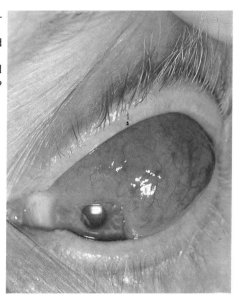

237 (a)Study the visual field anomaly and give the diagnosis.
(b)Given that the fields illustrated belong to the same patient and eye, which is the early stage?
(c)List other diagnostic tests that may be useful.

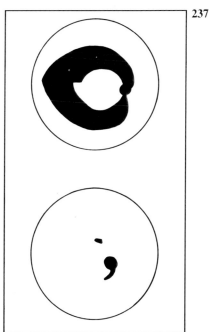

238

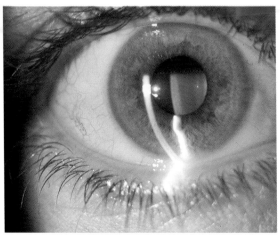

238 (a)What is this condition?
(b)What value has photography in routine out-patient work?

239 (a)What is this condition?
(b)What is the most common systemic association?
(c)List the possible corneal complications.

239

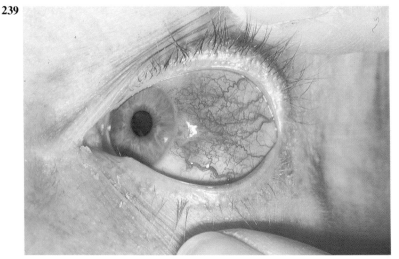

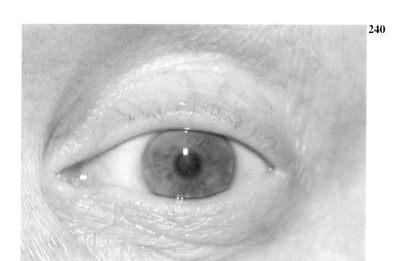

240,241 (a)Name this condition.
(b)Are there likely to be any eye/vision problems?

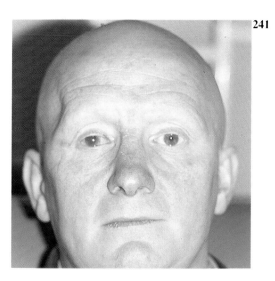

242

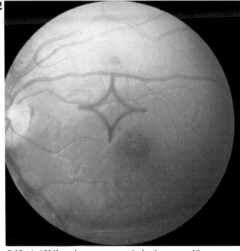

242 (a)What instrument is being used?
(b)The eye is fixating. What is the diagnosis?
(c)What is the treatment? Can normal vision result?

243 (a)Is this a rhegmatogeous detachment?
(b)What is the aetiology?
(c)What is the other eye likely to show?
(d)What is there to eliminate in the differential diagnosis?

243

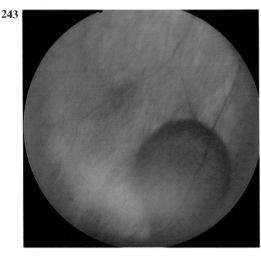

ANSWERS

1 (a)Choroid.
(b)Inflammatory—granulomatous choroiditis.
(c)Sympathetic ophthalmitis.

2 (a)Telescopic system (subnormal vision aid). The eye is made hyperopic with a -15.00 contact lens and the vision corrected by a $+10.50$ spectacle lens placed 30 mm from the cornea.
(b)To correct aniseikonia causing binocular vision problems.

3,4 (a)Infective keratitis (corneal ulcer).
(b)Endothelial dysgenesis, corneal dystrophies. Endothelial tears, due to birth trauma. Trigeminal (V) nerve dysgenesis (illustrated).

5,6 (a)Terriens marginal keratodystrophy. A non-inflammatory primary keratolysis limited to the peripheral cornea external to Bowman's membrane. Hence the thinning and widening of this zone, with pallisades of superficial vessels (not pannus). This is often misdiagnosed as pellucid keratoconus, but keratometry, whilst irregular, does have a flat component.
(b)Contact lenses. Keratoplasty is not advised.
(c)Anteriorly this resembles arcus degeneration, but the slit-beam appearance is diagnostic of Terriens.

7 (a)Perforation of the cornea.
(b)Loss of anterior chamber, prolapse of iris, endophthalmitis.
(c)Loss of basement membrane after corneal injury. Severe infection, pseudomonas aeruginosa, *Pneumococcal* and Herpes simplex infection also cause lysis. Other causes include systemic disease such as rheumatoid arthritis and sarcoidosis, rapid drying of the cornea as occurs in debility or coma, and toxaemia.

8 (a)Hydrops of cornea (acute keratoconus).
(b)Rupture of endothelial layer and descemes membrane with secondary Stromal oedema.
(c)Gradual decrease of oedema and improved vision in some cases. (Without a slit-beam microscope the frontal appearance is similar to desmetocoele.)

9 (a)Neurotrophic keratitis. An exposure keratitis due to anaesthesia of the cornea which permits trauma and desiccation of the cornea without reflex protection. There may also be lid levator paresis (Neuroparalytic keratitis).
(b)V trigeminal and VII facial nerves.
(c)Tarsorrhaphy, artificial tears.

10 (a)No. It is a gel contact lens surface drying phenomenon, with

proteo-lipid deposits on the lens.
(b)Keratoconjunctivitis sicca, corneal vascularisation, ulceration and
scarring. A filamentous keratitis is characteristic. Lacrimal gland
enlargement may occur.
(c)Rheumatoid arthritis, SLE, scleroderma, polyarteritis nodosa,
polymyositis, Hashimoto's disease, chronic hepatobiliary disease.

11 (a)Conjunctival naevus, (b)Pigmented conjunctival papilloma, malignant melanoma, granuloma pyogenicum, haemorrhagic lymphangioma.
(c)Observation and periodical photography.

12 (a)Herpes simplex (type 1) keratitis, dendritic phase showing typical
ulceration.
(b)Primary.
(c)Superficial keratitis, lid follicles, conjunctivitis, general malaise, fever,
adenitis.

13 (a)Corneal band degeneration, iris atrophy (secondary to chronic
uveitis).
N.B. Patient is wearing a contact lens to correct irregular astigmatism and
aphakia.
(b)Stills disease.
(c)Hyperparathyroidism, degenerate phthisical eyes, sarcoid, myeloma,
necrotic cornea from any cause with subsequent healing.

14 (a)Traumatic aniridia, coloboma of the lid.
(b)Photophobia.

15,16 (a)The pale fundus is the carrier and the pigmented fundus is a
pathological state of retinal epithelial pigment hypertrophy. In this
instance the morphology is pepper-and-salt distribution. This carrier
fundus does not show white radiating streaks from the macular area.
(sometimes seen in carriers).
(b)The visual disturbance for the pigmented fundus was constricted visual
fields and marked decrease of rod sensory function as determined by
history of night-blindness and electrodiagnostic tests. The carrier has
subnormal responses to electrical diagnostic tests, but no subjective
abnormality.

17 (a)Peter's anomaly. Posterior embryotoxon, dyscoria, Axenfeld's
syndrome, Reiger's anomaly.
(b)Glaucoma.

18 (a)Cortical cataract showing the suture lines posteriorly:
Fleischer-type cataract.
(b)There is no known association.

19,20 (a)Goldenhar's syndrome (oculo-auricular dysplasia).
(b)Epibulbar dermoid, accessory auricular appendage, mandibulo-facial
dysostosis, vertebral anomalies, skull anomalies,
lid coloboma, orbital tumours, Duane's retraction syndrome.

21 (a)The macula has no foveal reflex and a slight pigmentary epithelial anomaly.
(b)The amblyopia could be either central or peripheral in origin.

22 (a)Cystic degeneration of the stroma.
(b)Marfan's syndrome, Down's syndrome, atopic dermatitis, Apert syndrome.
(c)Fleischer pigment ring, acute hydrops, Bowman's membrane ruptures with superficial scarring, apical thinning, vernal conjunctivitis.

23,24 (a)Marcus–Gunn syndrome.
(b)A congenital anomalous cranial nerve synkinesis involving the trigeminal and oculomotor nerves.
(c)An exaggeration of a normally existing physiological co-contraction due to a congenital brain stem lesion.
(d)Usually becomes less conspicuous, and may resolve completely.

25 Infective keratitis, pannus, limbal pit (Herbert). Diagnosis: sub-acute trachoma (chlamydial infection).

26 (a)Papillary conjunctivitis with follicles.
(b)This papillary conjunctivitis is not vernal, but contact-lens trauma induced. Possibly due to altered proteins on the lens surface or preservatives in contact lens solutions.

27 (a)Localised areas of venous dilatation (not therefore a branch or total central retinal vein occlusion), vascular looping at disc (suggests some long-standing disc occlusion of retinal vein), exudation areas still evident.
(b)The most likely diagnosis is an inflammatory vasculitis. Differential diagnosis: arteriosclerosis (not marked in this fundus),
blood dyscrasias, retro-orbital disease, glaucoma.

28 (a)Developmental. Medullated fibres are not present in the newborn, but may develop after birth.
(b)A scotoma may be present.
(c)Optic atrophy or demyelination disease will decrease the medullation.

29,30 (a)Pseudo-disc oedema.
(b)Disc drusen (illustrated), hyaline bodies, myelinated fibres, hypoplastic disc, elevated disc (congenital).
(c)Transient visual disturbance can occur. Haemorrhages have been reported at disc head.

31 (a)Disc oedema and enlarged cilio-retinal vessel.
(b)This is the tapetum of a bovine eye.

32 (a)Malignant melanoma.
(b)Rare in black people.
(c)Retinal detachment, glaucoma, (anaesthesia of cornea), (neovascularisation).

33 (a)Cavernous haemangioma. The scan showed a circumscribed mass.

(b)Epidermal and dermoid cysts, teratomas, meningocele, mucocele, parasitic cysts (eg Echinococcus), other vascular neoplasms.

34 (a)Deep interstitial keratitis.
(b)Occurs in congenital syphilis. More common in males (61 per cent). Serological tests for syphilis were positive in this case.
(c)Band keratopathy, keratoconus, secondary glaucoma, ghost vessels.

35 (a)Basal cell carcinoma (less likely to be adenocarcinoma).
(b)Rarely.

36 (a)Diabetes mellitus.
(b)Venous dilatation, venous beading, venous loops, haemorrhages—dot and splinter. (c)Sub-internal limiting membrane haemorrhage, retinal oedema, cystoid macular oedema, exudates (post-proliferative—retinitis proliferans).

37 (a)It is eccentric to the vision line, giving gross irregular astigmatism.
(b)Immune graft rejection, vascularisation of cornea, astigmatism, macular oedema, cataract.

38 (a)A muco-epithelial tag in a dry eye.
(b)Sjögren's syndrome: xerostomia and keratoconjunctivitis sicca associated with a connective tissue disorder. Most commonly rheumatoid arthritis.

39 (a)Wegeners granulomatosis. It is characterised by a necrotising vasculitis and granulomatous inflammation affecting the respiratory tract and kidneys. Skin rashes are common. Half of patients have eye manifestation: iritis, scleritis and conjunctivitis are common. Retrobulbar granulomatous inflammation may cause exophthalmos.
(b)Immunosuppressive agents: cyclophosphamide, methotrexate, azathioprine, occasionally lobectomy for pulmonary lesions. Steroids are usually ineffective.

40 (a)The slide shows a tumour composed of mixed glandular and connective tissue elements. Benign mixed tumour.
(b)Lid swelling, tearing, pain, visual disturbance, limitation of motion.

41 (a)Artificial.
(b)This is a black occlusive contact lens which can be used for: insuperable diplopia, treatment of amblyopia, treatment of severe photophobia or prosthetic.

42 (a)Congenital dyscoria (possibly cleavage syndrome of anterior chamber—mesodermal dysgenesis, eg Reiger's syndrome).
(b)May be associated with microcornea, glaucoma, chorioretinal coloboma, cataract and lens dislocation.
(c)No treatment to improve vision is possible unless a cataract is present and matures.

43 (a)Chemical burn of the lower fornix.
(b)This will heal with deep fibrosis and loss of the fornix, symblepharon,

and dry eye complications of cornea.

44 (a)A nuclear cataract.
(b)Hardening and increasing pigmentation with ageing.
(c)Myopic shift in refraction resulting in improved near-vision.

45 Could be systemic disease treated by high-dosage anti-inflammatory drugs, concurrent infection, dry eye, graft rejection, immune deficiency or imperfect mechanical seal.

46 (a)Cystic dystrophy: basement membrane disease of Cogan.
(b)Usually asymptomatic, may get foreign body sensation due to erosions.
(c)Good.

47 (a)Keratoconus (Fleischer ring) due to haemosiderin deposition.
(b)Hudson–Stahli line, physiological trauma; Kayser–Fleischer ring, hepatolenticular degeneration; Stocker line, pterygium; Ferry line, anterior to a filtering bleb; pigment migration lines, melanin; heavy metals (eg silver, gold, iron, copper).

48 (a)Mydriasis, enophthalmos, heterochromic irides, ptosis, blepharophimosis.
(b)This shows Perry–Romberg syndrome.

49 Physiological cupping: C/D = 0.5.

50 Superficial keratitis is of several types. Central and above locations, Thygeson's epidemic keratoconjunctivitis; Inferior 1/3, staphylococcal blepharo-keratoconjunctivitis; superior limbal, chlamydial and palpebral conjunctivitis; central and palpebral fissure, exposure and neuropathic. This is a slide of contact-lens induced microdendritic, mosaic, isolated keratitis.

51 Endothelial separation (and folds) with stromal oedema.

52 (a)Macular dystrophy: Groenouw type II.
(b)Autosomal recessive, although most corneal dystrophies are transmitted as autosomal dominant defects.

53,54 (a)Bilateral oculomotor nerve paresis, myotonic dystrophy, myasthenia gravis, progressive external ophthalmoplegia, Eaton–Lambert syndrome.
(b)Skull X-ray, chest X-ray, tensilon test, thyroid function, anti-acetylcholine receptor antibodies, VDRL (serological syphilis test).

55,56 (a)Retrolental fibroplasia. Premature birth treated with high-concentration O_2. The retina shows neovascularisation and mesenchymal peripheral shunt zones (where there is avascular tissue), possibly related to a phase III condition of retrolental fibroplasia.
(b)Myopia, retinal pigmentation, vitreous membranes, heterotopia of the fovea, retinal detachments, cystoid macular oedema, cataract, glaucoma.
(c)Persistant hyperplastic primary vitreous, retinoblastoma, familial exudative vitreoretinopathy.

57 (a)Squamous cell epithelioma.
(b)Solar radiation damage may result in actinic keratosis, a pre-invasive lesion (more likely in fair-skinned individuals).
(c)Adequate surgical excision.

58 (a)The picture is that of cotton wool spot retinopathy (septic retinitis).
(b)When the cotton wool spots are due to a systemic bacteraemia, the centre of the spots are usually haemorrhagic in the infective phase (Roth spots). This is seen in subacute bacterial endocarditis. A similar retinal picture can be seen in HIV infection aetiology (sometimes related to generalised lymphadenopathy), and also pernicious anaemia.
(c)Serology and blood cultures to give aetiology of infective agent.

59 (a)Keratitis, conjunctivitis, photophobia, tearing.
(b)Cicatricial lid exposure keratitis, dry eye (mucus goblet cell atrophy), vaso-obliterative retinopathy, cataracts, hypoplastic deformities of bone.

60 (a)Senile (involutional) ectropia of lower lid and rhinophymatous nose.
(b)Laxity of the tarsoligamentous sling.
(c)Epiphora in patients with adequate tears, exposure symptoms in patients with deficient tears.

61,62 A hysterical ptosis, the blepharospasm being increased on any attempt to raise the lid. The lid is wrinkled due to contraction of orbicularis.

63,64 (a)A scleral lens with a ledge.
(b)Cataracts; external ophthalmoplegia (drugs had no local effect); baldness; face, neck and limb myopathy; testicular atrophy; retinal pigment epithelial dystrophy.

65 (a)Retinal epithelial hypertrophy, and this distribution is known as 'bear track'.
(b)Bear track retinal pigment is non-pathological. Conversely, corpuscular-type pigment associated with a retinal vessel distribution is likely to be intra-epithelial and pathological.

66 (a)Atopic eczema.
(b)Lid immobility can lead to drying of the cornea, with secondary disease of scarring, keratosis and vascularisation. Conjunctival papillitis is also seen. Cataract is common in atopic eczema (this may be steroid-induced).

67 Plica-semilunaris infection.

68 (a)True pterygium (involves the limbus).
(b)Basophilic degeneration (degeneration of sub-epithelial collagen), dissolution of Bowman zone of cornea, dyskeratatic epithelial cells, overlying the pterygium.
(c)Surgery: excision and anti-inflammatory drugs, dry eye treatment.

69 Epithelial cyst (trauma with inclusion cyst, miotic drugs), epithelial hyperplasia, epithelioma, embryonal tumour, malignant melanoma, neuronal tumour, leiomyoma. (This cyst does transilluminate, and is a benign epithelial cyst.)

70 (a)Central colloidal degeneration (Drusen).
(b)Hyaline excrescences on Bruch's membrane. If less discrete and more granular, may be lipid deposition from retinal pigment degeneration.

71,72 (a)Marfan's syndrome (dystrophia mesodermis congenita).
(b)Subluxed crystalline lens, arched palate, arachnodactyly, cardiovascular defects, keratoconus.
(c)Autosomal dominant.

73 (a)Right superior quadrantanopia with macular sparing. The presence of macular sparing strongly suggests a lesion of the occipital cortex, cerebrovascular disease or space-occupying lesion such as a tumour. Had the quadrantanopia been complete, then a lesion in the geniculo-calcarine radiation (Meyer loop) in the region of the temporal lobe should also be considered. Macular sparing may be the result of incomplete cortical neuronal destruction or due to shifts in ocular fixation.
(b)Full neurological work up may include CAT scan and NMR. Angiography may also be advised.

74 Retinal epithelial atrophy with granular lipid degeneration.

75 (a)Melanoma of palpebral conjunctiva.
(b)Treatment can be lid section or radiotherapy. Plastic surgery to protect the eye.

76 Chemical or thermal burn causing symblepharon.

77 (a)Yeast (*Candida albicans*) infection of keratoplasty. Note the colour and matt appearance typical of *Candida* infections.
(b)*Candida* infections commonly occur in eyes with decreased host defences: eg following keratoplasty, exposure keratitis, *Herpes simplex* keratitis, chronic use of steroids, keratitis sicca.

78 (a)Stevens–Johnson syndrome (erythema multiforma).
(b)Sulphonamides, penicillins, salicylates, topical anaesthetics, acetazolamide, phenytoin.

79 (a)Allergic—phlyctenular keratoconjunctivitis (illustrated);
Infective—keratoconjunctivitis, eg chlamydial; acne rosacea keratoconjunctivitis.
(b)Respectively, confirm palpebral conjunctival papillitis and folliculitis, eosinophilia in tears (allergy); late signs (pannus and Arlt's line) and microbiology (trachoma); history and facial signs.

80 (a)Optic disc pit.
(b)No, usually infero-temporal.
(c)Macular detachment in the adult.

81 Choroidal metastases, optic nerve atrophy.

82 (a)4/5 (0.8).
(b)Yes.
(c)Glaucomatous cupping with edge lipping. Disc pallor undermining, nasal shift of major retinal vessels, exposure of the lamina cribosa.

83 (a)Anterior uveitis with posterior synechiae.
(b)Trauma, causing iris prolapse; congenital, coloboma; surgical, iridectomy and intra-ocular lens implant, neurological eg., Horners Syndrome. Argyll-Robinson pupil; Drugs with central and peripheral mimetic action.

84 Breast and lung.

85 (a)Ectopia lentis.
(b)Trauma, Marfan's syndrome, Ehlers–Danlos syndrome, aniridia, Sturge–Weber syndrome, Weill–Marchesani syndrome, idiopathic, luetic, homocystinuria, buphthalmos, Crouzon disease, Spengel deformity, high myopia, congenital, hypermature cataract.
(c)Astigmatism, monocular diplopia, cataracts, iridodonesis. Anterior dislocation may cause glaucoma. Posterior dislocation will cause aphakia and may give rise to a chronic iritis or chorioretinal degeneration.

86 (a)Iridocyclitis, episcleritis, conjunctivitis, hypopyon.
(b)Reiter's syndrome, Behcet's disease, gonococcal arthritis, rheumatoid disease.

87 (a)Candle wax drippings.
(b)Sarcoidosis.
(c)Lymph node biopsy.
(d)Snowball vitreous infiltrates, uveitis, chorioretinal nodules, macula oedema, papilloedema, optic neuritis and secondary atrophy, lacrimal gland enlargement, extra-ocular muscle palsies, band keratopathy (hypercalcaemia).

88 (a)Nummular keratitis.
(b)Brucella, *Escherichia coli*, viral.

89 Fatty infiltration with feeding vessel.

90 (a)Stromal plastic implant for bullous keratopathy.
(b)It has been performed using gas-permeable material to correct high myopia.

91 (a)'Bull eye' maculopathy—perifoveal retina is hypopigmented.
(b)Fenestrated sheen macular dystrophy (autosomal dominant) and progressive cone–rod dystrophy and chloroquine retinopathy give similar appearances.

92 Toxic keratitits due to preservative in ophthalmic preparation.

93 Filtration for treatment of glaucoma. (Note also the graft previously done because of scarring secondary to trachoma.)

94 (a)Leber's optic atrophy. Sex-linked inheritance.
(b)Oedematous.

(c)Swollen nerve fibres.

95 (a)Mesodermal dysplasia, birth injury, hyaline reduplication from Descemet's membrane.
(b)Bullous keratopathy.

96,97 (a)Diro-filaria repens—a nematode infection 100mm long and much larger than the *Loa loa* type.
(b)Africa. Infected female deer-fly is commonly quoted for loa loa but this worm has dog as primary host. Ingestion from contaminated water.
(c)Eosinophilia, parasite in a thick blood smear.
(d)Yes, diethyl carbamizine.

98 (a)Leprosy.
(b)Early signs: corneal nerve beading, iris pearls; late signs: chalky corneal deposits and evidence of anterior uveitis.

99 (a)Retinal digest preparation, showing eosinophilic degeneration of the pericyte nucleus.
(b)The significance of the pericyte change is unknown but it may be a factor in microaneurysm formation. (see **36**).

100 (a)Retinoblastoma.
(b)Flexner–Wintersteiner rosettes.
(c)Deletion of the long arm of chromosome 13.

101 (a)Granular keratodystrophy, Groenouw's type.
(b)Picture **52**.

102,103 (a)Yes, this is Axenfeld's syndrome—anterior displacement of Schwalbe's line.
(b)Yes, a form of posterior embryotoxon.
(c)Glaucoma.

104 (a)Dermoid at the limbus.
(b)May be excised, followed by occasional use of a prosthetic contact lens; may require an annular graft; or may be left alone.

105,106 (a)The left macular is atrophic: the diagnosis was a rod–cone dystrophy. (Note also the tigroid fundi.)
(b)Diminished acuity, field defects, colour vision anomaly.

107 It is a phase-interference picture of the tear film. Anterior specular micropscopy can show this and also polarised light.

108 Posterior lens cortex. Subcapsular steroid-induced cataract with vacuoles.
109 (a)Posterior keratoconus with lenticonus.
(b)Congenital.
(c)None.

110 Keratoconus.

111 (a)Buphthalmos (infantile glaucoma).
(b)Angle trabeculae anomaly, endothelial dysfunction, epithelial and

stromal oedema with ulceration and recurrent infections, corneal vascularisation and scarring.

112 (a)Episcleral venous engorgement–congestion.
(b)Carotid–venous fistula, pulsating exophthalmos ocular bruit, diplopia, headache, conjunctival chemosis and superior ophthalmic vein 'arteriolisation' with venous congestion (illustrated).
(c)Cavernous carotid and cavernous sinus, more rarely meningeal carotids (anastomosis with exterior carotid, interior carotid and vertebral arteries) and cavernous sinus tributaries.
(d)Developmental arteriovenous malformation (a tortuous mass of arteries and veins with no capillary bed). Mass has neurological localising signs such as mental change, visual tract lesions, hemispherical signs, CAT scan diagnosis. No history of trauma.

113 (a)Macular star.
(b)Severe hypertension, often of renal origin.
(c)The deposits are distributed in Henle's layer, which is elongated and oblique around the macula, thus giving a radial appearance.

114 (a)Radial keratotomy.
(b)Overcorrection (poor technique), fluctuation of acuity, irregular astigmatism, glare and flare, recurrent erosions, epithelial downgrowth, penetration of A.C., infection.

115,116 (a)Iris sphincter atrophy. Iridectomies.
(b)Uretz–Zavalla syndrome: first reported as induced by cycloplegiacs, after keratoplasty with associated hypertension.

117 (a)Desmetocoele of keratoplasty from supurative keratitis.
(b)*Pseudomonas aeruginosa* infection.

118 (a)Dyskeratosis and leukoplakia, occlusion of Meibomian orifices, trichiasis, blepharitis, secondary corneal vascularisation.
(b)Stevens–Johnson syndrome (Erythema multiforme).
(c)A diffuse immune vasculitis with a prominence of eosinophils and lymphocytes. There is a deposition of complexes of circulating antigen with complement fixing antibodies.

119 (a)Fuchs dystrophy: endothelial cell dysfunction.
(b)Keratodystrophies involving endothelium, mesodernal dysplasias, trauma and physicochemical insult, vitreous contact, uveitis, contact lens anoxia.

120 (a)Oculo-cutaneous albinism.
(b)Nystagmus, decreased acuity, increased incidence of strabismus and astigmatism, macular hyperplasia, visible choroidal vasculature.
(c)Tinted contact lenses may reduce nystagmoid movement, and can be of prosthetic value.
(d)Psychological problems, predisposition to ultraviolet-induced cutaneous neoplasms.

121,122 (a)Melanoma of choroid (note any lipofuschin areas, retinal detachment and haemorrhage), naevus, choroidal haemorrhage, subretinal

hyaline membrane haemorrhage, senile pigmentary central epithelial degeneration, histoplasmosis infection (typically shows atrophic choroid and pigment deposition).
(b)Polygonal cells with abundant cytoplasm, conspicuous nucleus, some melanin ie., melanoma of epithelioid cell type.

123 (a)A lymphatic hyperplasia: B-cell lymphoma.
(b)Late systemic involvement is rare.

124–126 (a)Deep corneal opacities, cherry red macula, retinitis pigmentosa.
(b)Mucopolysaccharide syndrome (MPS 11)—Hunter's syndrome.
(c)Dermatan and heparin sulphate. (Hurler's syndrome has a similar clinical picture, but is more severe.)
(d)X-linked. All other MPS syndromes are autosomal recessive.

127 Buphthalmos (glaucoma, stromal oedema, a painful condition), megalocornea (male, clear cornea).

128 (a)Basal cell carcinoma.
(b)They account for 80–90 per cent of malignant lid tumours, and 20 per cent of all lid tumours.

129 Chronic granuloma of Meibomian gland. Section shows macrophages and giant cells surrounded by lymphocytes and plasma cells with lipoid granules.

130 It is a pre-cancerous melanoma of the conjunctiva.

131 (a)Anophthalmos may be bilateral. It is usually associated with other developmental abnormalities.
(b)Orbital implants and/or prosthesis. After puberty plastic surgery may be beneficial.

132 Yes. Gunshot powder tattooing of conjunctiva.

133 Inclusion iris filtration operation (now obsolete).

134,135. (a)Osteogenesis imperfecta.
(b)An autosomal dominant condition.
(c)Associated with a deficiency in collagen production.
(d)They include thinning of the sclera (giving blue colour), corneal arcus, keratoconus, megalocornea, marginal corneal thinning, hyperopia.

136 (a)Blood staining (haemosiderin) of the posterior cornea.
(b)It occurred following a total hyphaemia caused by concussion injury, which precipitated a secondary glaucoma due to angle block.

137 Scleromalacia (the other eye is likely to be affected and a history of rheumatoid disease elicited), choroidal melanoma (intraocular involvement is likely), ruptured sclera.

138 (a)High myopia.
(b)Temporal crescent*, posterior staphyloma*, incipient glaucoma, choroidal atrophy*, Bruch's membrane clefts (lacquer cracks*), Fuchs

macular black spot (choroidal haemorrhage); lattice degeneration of retina, retinal holes and tears, vitreous detachment, vitreous degeneration with floaters. (*Illustrated.)

139 (a)Pre-chiasmal lesion involving left optic nerve and chiasma.
(b)Foster–Kennedy syndrome.. A sub-frontal mass could cause optic atrophy on one side (of the lesion), and papilloedema is then only seen in the non-atrophic disc (enlarged disc scotoma — illustrated).

140 (a)Epikeratoprosthesis (forerunner of epikeratoplasty techniques).
(b)Aphakic bullous keratopathy—it relieves pain and improves vision.
(c)Stromal vascularisation, infection, growth of epithelium beneath lens causing it to become dislodged.

141,142 (a)Graves dysthyroid orbitopathy associated with exophthalmos, conjunctival oedema and hyperaemia, lower scleral gap, extra-ocular muscle myopathy, decreased blink rate and absence of forehead wrinkles.
(b)The pupil is dilated secondary to an optic nerve lesion.

143 (a)A connective tissue disorder, the features of which include: tight firm skin, Raynaud's phenomenon, subcutaneous calcification, oesphageal hypomotility, malabsorption, pulmonary fibrosis, cardiomyopathy and renal failure.
(b)Eye complications include dry eye and trichiasis, and melting cornea (as in the picture).

144 (a)An old adult.
(b)Loss of goblet cells.
(c)Benign mucous membrane atrophy (ocular pemphigoid).

145,146 (a)Sclero-keratitis.
(b)Since the aetiology is the same as for the episcleritis they tend to repond to the same treatment, and if treated early enough permanent changes may be avoided. However, some degree of permanent scarring often remains.

147,148 (a)Angio-neurotic oedema. May be due to deficiency of C_1 Esterase Inhibitor (autosomal dominant).
(b)Allergy to insect bites, contact lens solutions or cosmetics may produce a similar picture, but resolution would be delayed.

149 This patient has Moebius syndrome. It is possible, but much less likely that the patient has a coincident Duane's retraction syndrome, congenital esotropia, or hypoplastic lateral recti with 7th nerve palsy.

150 The choroid. This is juxtapapillary choroiditis (Jensen). It is not disc oedema. Histoplasmosis infection should be considered.

151 (a)Angioid streaks: cracks in the collagenous and elastic portion of Bruch's membrane.
(b)Collagen disorders and other conditions: pseudo-xanthoma elasticum, Ehlers–Danlos syndrome, Paget's disease, sickle cell anaemia, acromegaly, lead poisoning, hypercalcaemia.

152 (a)Terson's syndrome: vitelline membrane at the disc associated with haemorrhage.
(b)Corneal oedema, retinal detachment, cataract, recurrent haemorrhage.
(c)Neovascular glaucoma retinal detachment, cataract, recurrent haemorrhage (in diabetes), haemolytic and erythroclastic glaucoma.

153 Congenital. It is a coloboma of the macula. The choroid shows no evidence of an inflammatory reaction.

154–156 (a)Yes, they are all eyes with retinoblastoma. **154** Very early 'fatty' change in retina; **155**, pigmented arcus and some calcium refractile spots; **156** white pupillary reflex ('cat's eye' reflex) of advanced stage.
(b)Differential diagnosis at the later stage includes: toxacara, Coat's disease, uveitis, retrolental fibroplasia, persistent hyperplastic vitreous organisation of neonatal retinal haemorrhage, juvenile retinoschisis and toxoplasmosis.

157 (a)'Morning glory' disc.
(b)A congenital coloboma of the disc or glial tissue of the disc head.
(c)Congenital forebrain anomalies including basal encephalocele.

158 Acne rosacea with associated keratitis shows limbal infiltration with progressive sector vascularisation and scarring. Demodex folliculorum is often found in a skin biopsy of the nose or eyelid.

159,160 (a)Leukoplakia (dyskeratosis) of conjunctiva (**159**), of cornea (**160**) due to tear deficiency (see **118**).
(b)Leukoplakia is a clinical, and thus descriptive, term, and on microscopic examination may reveal pseudo-epitheliomatous dysplasias, carcinamas *in situ* or even invasive cancer.

161 (a)Amoeboid ulceration of cornea. Shows heaped up epithelium and stromal involvement.
(b)Indolent ulceration, stromal keratitis, bacterial superinfection, toxicity to antiviral agents with secondary keratopathy.

162,163 (a)Fuchs primary endothelial dystrophy (Guttata). The endothelial cells have flat excrescences giving rise to the typical 'beaten metal' appearance.
(b)Dehydration preparations, eg 5 per cent sodium chloride drops and ointment, may help to reduce epithelial oedema. A soft bandage contact lens will decrease discomfort caused by rupture of epithelial bullae.

164,165 (a)Herpes zoster ophthalmicus.
(b)Eyelid, conjunctival and corneal vesicles; keratitis; uveitis (common); optic atrophy (rare); post-herpetic neuralgia and keratoneuropathy (165); episcleritis; muscle palsies, secondary glaucoma.

166 Penetrating keratoprosthesis (Cardona type). Used for opaque cornea when keratoplasty is not possible (rejection, dry eye). A Choyce type buried keratoprosthesis is probably better for dry eye.

167 (a)No. It is persistant pupillary membrane (dilated pupil to illustrate

anomaly).
(b)It does not interfere with vision.

168 (a)Congential epicapsular pigment stars.
(b)Yes.
(c)Remnants of the anterior tunica vasculosa.

169,170 The complication was hypoparathyroidism with consequential hypocalcaemia. Ca^{2+} ions are essential for corneal metabolism—note the sub-epithelial clouding.

171 (a)Mooren's ulcer. Note lipping at inner edge.
(b)Thought to be auto-immune in origin, as antibodies to corneal epithial antigens have been isolated.

172 (a)Rhegmatogenous retinal detachment (old, untreated).
(b)Vitreous traction, retinal degeneration, trauma, also developmental factors such as myopia and Marfan's syndrome, retinal vascular disorders, neoplasm, metabolic disease.

173 Congenital cystic anomaly of endothelium.

174 (a)Keratoglobus.
(b)Needs no surgical treatment, only a scleral contact lens.

175 Iris coloboma. A congenital condition.

176 (a)Pterygium.
(b)Dry, dusty, sunny environments.

177 (a)Mascara tattooing (cosmetic).
(b)Adrenochrome, from use of adrenaline; yellow discoloration, jaundice, excess carotene, ochronosis, Addision's disease, naevi.

178 Gold or platinum tattooing to simulate a pupil.

179 Endothelial plaques (possibly fibrous tissue).

180 (a)Facial nerve.
(b)(Bell's palsy) with a secondary exposure keratitis.

181 (a)Transillumination.
(b)This would differentiate between a solid tumour and a cystic lesion.

182 Naevus, lymphangioma, capillary angioma (this was proven by histology).

183 (a)Toxocara infection (nematode).
(b)Unilateral endophthalmitis, strabismus, leukocoria. These are often associated with a history of close contact with dogs, cats or pica.
(c)Skin testing, blood eosinophilia, serology.

184 (a)Central serous retinopathy.
(b)60 per cent recover is 3 months, in 20 per cent the disease lasts more than 6 months. A benign self-limiting disease.
(c)Usually no treatment, as the condition is self-limiting, but laser photocoagulation can be used in long-standing cases.

185 Retinal detachment, showing a degenerative retina.

186 Bowen's disease (intra-epithelial epithelioma).

187 (a)Senile ectatic conjunctival fold covering the lower limbus.
(b)No.

188 (a)Blunt trauma.
(b)Berlin's oedema.
(c)The inflammatory reponse is sub-retinal at this stage.

189 (a)These are not white cells, but asteroid hyalosis bodies. The patient is aphakic, thus the vitreous is in the anterior chamber.
(b)Remnant of lens capsule.
(c)None.
(d)Calcium soaps.

190 Haemangioma, rhabdomyosarcoma, retinoblastoma, neuroblastoma, orbital cyst, glioma of optic nerve, lymphoma, sarcoma (undifferentiated).

191 (a)Zonular cataract.
(b)It can be hereditary, often being autosomal dominant, and bilateral.

192 (a)Rubella cataract. The right eye has a white plaque type and the left eye a nuclear cataract.
(b)The maternal rubella syndrome consists of cataract, nerve deafness, mental retardation and cardiac lesions (typically PDA, septal defects).
An extended syndrome exists involving other body systems.

193 (a)Histoplasmosis.
(b)Choroidal histo spot. Hypertrophic parafoveal scarring is pathognomic, but is not seen here.
(c)Neonatal infection, jaundice and encephalitis, acute febrile illness of lympho-adenopathic form.

194 (a)Heterochromia iridis.
(b)Heterochromia iridum, Horner's syndrome, Fuchs heterochromic cyclitis, Waadenburg–Klein syndrome.

195 Penetrating glass injury. A glass splinter can be seen in the anterior chamber (6 o'clock).

196 (a)Anterior staphylomata of cornea in an adult, due to corneal perforation in infancy secondary to an exanthem.
(b)Phthis, choroidal melanoma.

197 (a)Congenital microphthalmia.
(b)May occur alone or be associated with chromosomal abnormalities, congenital rubella, toxoplasmosis, etc.
(c)Treatment is with a prosthetic shell.

198 (a)Blurred disc outline, pink disc, engorged retinal veins, haemorrháges.
(b)Papilloedema.

199 (a)Angioid streaks, maculopathy.
(b)Pseudo-xanthoma elasticum, Paget's disease, Ehlers–Danlos syndrome, sickle-cell anaemia, lead poisoning, acromegaly. The streaks may also occur in normal individuals.

200 There is keratohyaline production in the prickle cell layer, giant tumour cells (with hypochromatic nuclei) and multi-nucleated cells. This can develop into squamous cell carcinoma.

201 (a)Hypertensive retinopathy.
(b)Vessel tortuosity, flame and blot haemorrhages, macular star, cotton wool spots.

202 Corneal perforation, secondary to exposure keratitis with trichiasis.

203 Ophthalmic drop sensitivity. Note only the skin is affected and not the eye itself—a contact dermatitis.

204 (a)Saltzmann's "keratodystrophy".
(b)A condition secondary to phlyctenular keratitis.

205 Bowen's dyskeratosis. The cells are oedematous, and vacuolated giant cells and giant tumour cells may be present.

206 (a)Lattice degeneration.
(b)Myopia.

207 Reis–Bucklers keratodystrophy. An autosomal dominant condition affecting chiefly the basement membrane and basal layer cells.

208,209 (a)Vernal catarrhal conjunctivitis (chronic), showing papillae with a heavy leucocytic invasion.
(b)Giant papilliary conjunctivitis induced by contact lens wear.

210 Penetrating keratoplasty, aphakia, hyphaema, vitreous adhesion to endothelium and localised Bullous keratopathy. General stromal oedema and vascularisation.

211 Naevus and Drusen bodies.

212 A demarcation line at the reattachment of a retinal detachment.

213,214 (a)Congenital. (No evidence of invasive trauma).
(b)Glaucoma.

215 (a)Retinitis Albescens — night vision poor — constricted fields of vision.
(b)Retinitis Pigmentosa.
(c)Electrodiagnostic tests.

216 It produces against-the-rule astigmatism (and therefore neutralises with-the-rule astigmatism common to circular grafts).

217,218 Yes. Congenital iris and chorioretinal coloboma.
Find another pupil dycoria in the text. Does it have the same aetiology?

219 Persistent hyaloid corkscrew vessel.

220 No.

221 An internuclear ophthalmoplegia—adduction failure with abduction nystagmus in the opposite eye.
(a)The lesion is in the median longitudinal bundle/fasciculus.
(b)It is most typical of multiple sclerosis.

222 Sub-internal limiting membrane haemorrhage and proliferative retinopathy (neovascularisation and vitreous involvement secondary to retinal hypoxia).

223 (a)Blue sclera.
(b)Normal at birth, osteogenesis imperfecta, Marfan's syndrome, myopia, rheumatoid arthritis, long-standing inflammation, oculo-mandibulo facial dyscephaly—Hallerman–Streiff syndrome, anterior keratoconus (allied to collagen deficiency), ageing.

224 (a)This patient wears a false right eye, small pupil size for day use and large pupil for night.
(b)Essential anisocoria—congenital, Horner's syndrome, tonic pupil (Holmes–Adie syndrome), Argyll–Robertson pupil (irregular and small), mid-brain lesion (depressed pupil reflexes and other neurological signs), atropine (fixed dilated and history of drops), IIIrd nerve palsy and associated extra-ocular muscle palsy.

225,226 Local and sinus pathology, pseudotumour, secondary tumours and lymphomas. Vascular and neural tumours are less likely.

227,228 Benign (naevus of retina).

229 (a)Hypertensive retinopathy.
(b)Grade I, arteriolar attenuation, early arterio-venous crossing changes; Grade II, marked arterio-venous crossing changes, areas of arteriolar constriction, hard exudates, linear haemorrhages; Grade III, retinal oedema, cotton wool patches, haemorrhages, copper wire-attenuation of vessels; Grade IV, as Grade III with papilloedema subhyaline haemorrhage, silver-wire attenuation of vessels. There are many variations of this classification.
(c)Grade III hypertensive retinopathy.

230,231 (a)Xenon-arc photocoagulation. The scarring and pigmentary burn reactions are typical. Laser burns are much smaller in diameter, and the depth of reaction depends on the wavelength and time period. A large range with selective functions is now available.
(b)A green filter, giving red-free light, helps to illustrate haemorrhages.

232 (a)The Drusen (colloid bodies of degenerate Bruch's membrane) are arranged in a circinate pattern. True circinate retinopathy.
(b)If associated with leaking vessels, as shown by angiofluorography, can be treated by laser therapy.

233 Coat's disease. Usually unilateral, a perivaculitic condition with leaking retinal vessels.

234 (a)Ophthalmomyiasis. The hypopigmented tracks are the pathways of larvae of the flies *Diptera*. The maggots bore their way into the eye.
(b)The sclera of a child is easier to penetrate than that of an adult.

235 Solar burn of macula—eclipse blindness.

236 (a)Conjunctival lymphoma.
(b)If the histology shows a reactive lymphocytic hyperplasia (B-cell type) and within the classification of pseudo B− tumour, then systemic involvement is unlikely.
(c)Systemic lymphoma—with orbital involvement, B-cell replication most common of a rare condition; leukaemias with orbital involvement are a more common association; pseudo-tumours and lacrimal tumours.

237 (a)Chronic simple glaucoma, blind-spot enlargement, arcuate scotoma.
(b)The lower (central field) is the early finding.
(c)Tonography, provocative tests, gonioscopy, optic disc evaluation, acuity and contrast sensitivity, colour vision anomalies, cardiovascular system (hypertension).

238 (a)Naevus of the iris.
(b)A photographic record is often more accurate than words; to follow-up progress, eg tumours; legal considerations.

239 (a)Episcleritis (nodule formation).
(b)Rheumatoid disease.
(c)Stromal infiltrates—especially lipid, limbal guttering, keratolysis, stromal keratitis.

240,241 (a)Alopecia.
(b)In the patient shown there were no eye/vision problems.
Vogt–Koyanagi–Harada syndrome and sympathetic ophthalmia can be associated with partial alopecia.

242 (a)Opthalmoscope fitted with a projected fixation target. Pleoptoscope.
(b)Small-angle strabismus, with fixation anomaly and amblyopia.
(c)Occlusion of the amblyopic eye, followed by foveal stimulation. Rotating blue polarised light, light ablation of the fixation zone followed by repetitive foveal stimulation. Treatment unlikely to be successful if the other eye has normal vision.

243 (a)This is a non-rhegmatogenous detachment (separation) of the retina. It transilluminates.
(b)Often called a cyst of the retina (congenital).
(c)A similar condition in exactly the same location, or residual evidence of separation.
(d)M.M. of choroid.